THE ESSENTIAL GUIDE TO

Home Herbal REMEDIES

Easy Recipes Using Medicinal Herbs to Treat More than **125** Conditions from Sunburns to Sore Throats

MELANIE WENZEL

Robert **ROSE**

G|U

Dedication: For Frank. Your healing power has done wonders for me

For complete cataloguing information, see page 248.

Disclaimer
This book is a general guide only and should never be a substitute for the skill, knowledge, and experience of a
qualified medical professional dealing with the facts, circumstances, and symptoms of a particular case.

The nutritional, medical, and health information presented in this book is based on the research, training, and
professional experience of the author, and is true and complete to the best of her knowledge. However, this book is
intended only as an informative guide for those wishing to know more about health, nutrition, and medicine; it is
not intended to replace or countermand the advice given by the reader's personal physician. Because each person and
situation is unique, the author and the publisher urge the reader to check with a qualified health-care professional
before using any procedure where there is a question as to its appropriateness. A physician should be consulted
before beginning any exercise program. The author and the publisher are not responsible for any adverse effects or
consequences resulting from the use of the information in this book. It is the responsibility of the reader to consult a
physician or other qualified health-care professional regarding his or her personal care.

The recipes or formulas in this book have been carefully tested. To the best of our knowledge, they are safe
and nutritious for ordinary use and users. For those people with food or other allergies, or who have special food
requirements or special health issues, please read the suggested contents of each recipe or formula carefully and
determine whether or not they may create a problem for you. All recipes or formulas are used at the risk of the
consumer.

We cannot be responsible for any hazards, loss or damage that may occur as a result of any recipe or formula used.

For those with special needs, allergies, requirements or health problems, in the event of any doubt, please contact
your medical adviser prior to the use of any recipe or formula.

Design and production: Martina Hwang/PageWave Graphics Inc.
Editor: Tina Anson Mine
Copy editor/proofreader: Austen Gilliland
Indexer: Beth Zabloski
Translator: Sylvia Goulding

Cover image: Kramp + Gölling, Hamburg

Interior photography: Dpa picture-alliance: p.12.
Kramp + Gölling, Hamburg: p.3–6, 9–10, 13–25, 30–31, 33–34, 48, 64, 82, 90, 100, 110, 122, 130, 140,
152–245
Astrid Obert, München: p.7–8, 29, 32, 36–47, 51–63, 67–81, 84–89, 93–99, 102–109, 113–121, 125–129,
133–139, 143–151.

The publisher gratefully acknowledges the financial support of our publishing program by the Government of
Canada through the Canada Book Fund.

Published by Robert Rose Inc.
120 Eglinton Avenue East, Suite 800, Toronto, Ontario, Canada M4P 1E2
Tel: (416) 322-6552 Fax: (416) 322-6936
www.robertrose.ca

Printed and bound in Canada

1 2 3 4 5 6 7 8 9 TCP 22 21 20 19 18 17 16 15 14

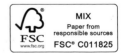

Contents

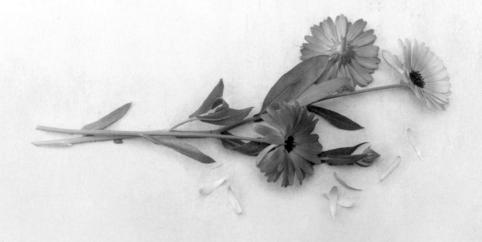

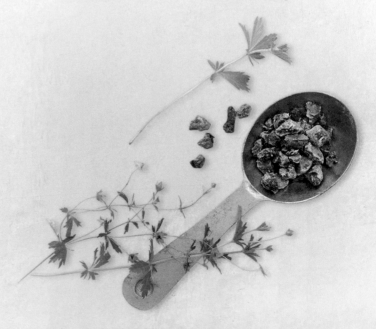

Preface

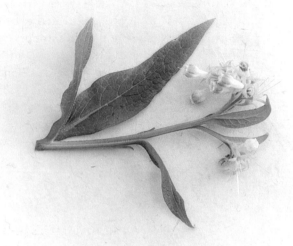

People's interest in gentle, low-cost remedies is getting stronger all the time. Alternative medicine, medicinal plants and herbs lost their frumpy, hippie image a long time ago. And people who are interested in natural health today certainly don't want to embark on a boring ideological argument about conventional versus alternative medicine. They just want to make use of long-standing, tried-and-tested treatments—possibly in combination with the range of cures offered by conventional medicine and the pharmaceutical and cosmetic industries.

Nature Is Cool

I was well placed to observe this trend. As a qualified, registered nonmedical practitioner, I have been running a classical homeopathy family practice for 12 years in Cologne, Germany. At the same time, I'm also the resident expert on medicinal plants for the TV series "At Home and on the Road," broadcast by WDR Television. In this position, the audience's reaction gives me an excellent feeling for the topics and issues that particularly interest people.

Over the last few years, I have been asked with increasing frequency which natural remedy might help with this ache or that medical complaint. And whoever asked always wanted the solution to be "only something very basic." At one point, I realized that there was a great demand for such "very basic" recipes—the ones that I was jotting down each time, every one of them just a few words on a piece of paper. That's how I came up with the idea of bringing all of these recipes together and writing this book.

The book is not aimed at readers who have been long-time followers of natural medicine. I wrote it especially for people who have not yet discovered the benefits of herbal medicine for themselves. I am hoping that they will develop a "taste" for it and realize how much fun and satisfaction there is in making these wonderful remedies at home.

Perhaps you're saying to yourself, "Well, these 'little remedies' from the natural pharmacy will, of course, only help for minor ailments." But you'd be wrong. Admittedly, for years, I was also rather skeptical about the efficacy of many natural remedies. I was particularly conscious of this fact during my pregnancies. Although I desperately wanted to treat one or another of my ailments in a gentle, natural way, at the same time I sighed and said to myself, "Well, it probably won't help a lot." It really is strange how much we are all marked by our belief that chemicals, although harmful in some ways, are nevertheless highly effective. But herbal medicine is as effective as, and no less important than, chemical products. That's why I felt it was important to show you in the Plant Portraits from A–Z section (page 154) what scientists say about the healing properties of and the applications for each plant.

My Recipes

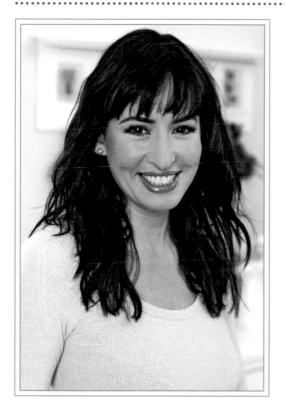

At the heart of this book are the home remedy recipes, which start on page 33. They are all highly effective, but not difficult or time-consuming to make. The ingredients are widely available, and you'll only need common kitchen utensils found in every household to make them. So if you're wondering what prior knowledge, skills or abilities you might need to make these remedies, the answer is none. There is nothing special required in order to work your way through these recipes—and there's no danger to life and limb. If you can cook spaghetti, you have all the experience you need to successfully follow the recipes in this book.

I hope with all my heart that you will be inspired by my enthusiasm for the world and the power of medicinal plants.

Kind regards,
Melanie Wenzel

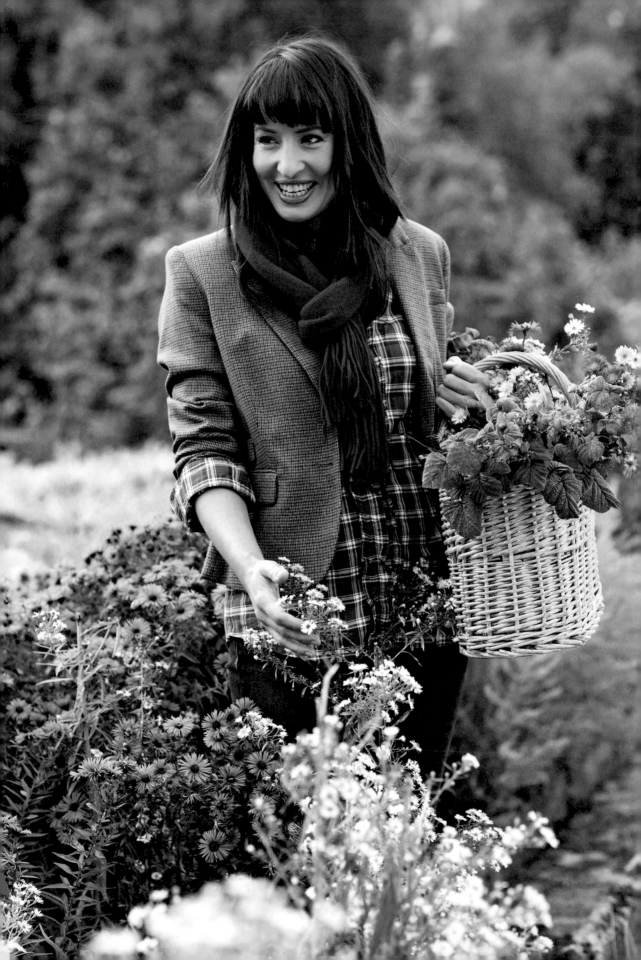

The Green Pharmacy

More and more people are returning to the centuries-old tradition of herbal medicine. After all, nature offers just as many effective remedies today as it did in times past. These remedies are successful at treating all sorts of illnesses—as well as the unpleasant side effects of modern life, including stress, exhaustion and listlessness. Even scientists have acknowledged that herbal medicine possesses an array of healing powers.

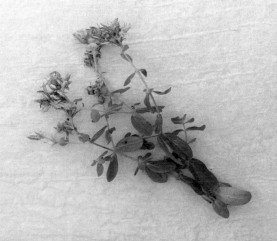

A Brief History of Herbal Medicine

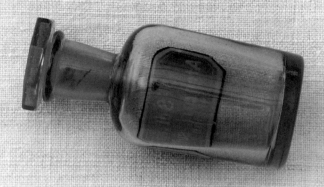

Like so many other things, the "natural pharmacy" almost disappeared into the darkness of history. As quickly as scientists have developed ever more drugs in past decades, common knowledge of the healing power of plants has slipped deeper and deeper into oblivion. This has happened despite the fact that, since time immemorial, people have used naturally occurring substances to strengthen their mental and physical well-being, and to treat and cure illnesses.

The Beginnings of Medicine

It is impossible to determine today who among our ancestors first used plants—or their active components, to be precise—for medicinal purposes. However, it is safe to assume that the idea is as old as humankind itself. At first, prehistoric humans probably simply followed their instincts, eating berries, chewing roots and placing leaves on the wounds they received. Among the items that Ötzi, the Neolithic (New Stone) or Chalcolithic (Copper) Age mummy who was discovered in a glacier in the Ötztal Alps in 1991, carried in his bag were fire-making tools, such as tinder and pyrite, plus a birch polypore fungus. Known for its anti-inflammatory action, the fungus continued to be used as a remedy for a long time, often for dressing wounds.

The more advanced civilization became, the more people understood about which plants could bring relief for what ailments. Initially, this knowledge was probably passed on orally, from one generation to the next. The oldest preserved written records date back to Babylonia. These clay tablets, which are more than 4,500 years old, contain records of the symptoms of and remedies for a variety of diseases. Several ancient Egyptian papyri are also valuable sources on the history of medicine. Thanks to them, we know that ancient Egyptians suffered from ailments that still impair the quality of life for countless people today, such as rheumatism and a variety of infectious diseases. Some of these scrolls also impart information on medical care at that time. The Ebers Papyrus, for example, which was discovered in Luxor at the end of the 19th century, contains many hundreds of formulas and remedies for decoctions, gargling solutions, inhalations, incense blends, pills and creams. Some of the plants in these recipes—such as castor plants and poppies—were used until modern times.

The Ancient World

After the decline of the Egyptian empire, knowledge of healing plants spread throughout the ancient world and influenced the medical knowledge of the Hebrews, Arabs, Persians, Greeks and Romans. The Greek physician Theophrastus of Eresus (372–287 BC), regarded as the "father" of botany, compiled the first complete work about the world of plants; the book is still preserved today. In the ninth volume of his *Enquiry into Plants,* Theophrastus also deals with drinks and remedies made from various plants, thus laying the foundation for pharmacology.

The medicinal knowledge of the ancient Greeks strongly influenced life and culture under the Roman Empire. Yet it was again a Greek man who advanced this knowledge. In his *De material medica,* the military physician Pedanius Dioscorides (AD 40–90)

described more than 600 plants and their uses. The book became the standard medical reference in Europe and was used right up to the early modern period. The methods for manufacturing medicines developed by the Roman physician Galen of Pergamon served physicians as the scientific basis for medical treatments into the 17th century.

Early Christendom

Unfortunately, much of this medicinal knowledge was lost to the common people with the rise of Christianity. The traditions were preserved only in Christian monasteries and abbeys; monastic physicians, pharmacies and hospitals administered this great wealth of medicinal knowledge in Europe. Just as today, we visit a doctor or pharmacist when we feel ill, in the past people went to a monastery in order to be treated or to buy a remedy. The members of these religious orders initially collected wild medicinal herbs— for their teas and tinctures, drops and ointments—in nearby woods and meadows. But soon they created their own gardens of medicinal plants within the monastery walls. In addition to indigenous plant species, they also grew plants that monks

Capitulare de Villis

....

In 812, Charlemagne (747–814) enacted a charter, or capitulary, called the *Capitulare de Villis Vel Curtis Imperialibus*. It stipulated which plants should be cultivated in the imperial estates and monasteries—a total of 73 useful plants and 16 trees—including medicinal herbs that are still popular today, such as marigold, mint, fennel, caraway, mallow, lemon balm (Melissa) and sage. His capitulary determined the layout of many cottage gardens, whose typical mixture of medicinal, culinary and ornamental plants is once again sought today. With this charter, Charlemagne also created the foundations of health care for his people.

In the past few decades, gardens planted in accordance with ancient rules have been recreated in many places. In Germany, there are Charlemagne's herb garden behind Aachen's city hall, the Karlsgarten west of Aachen, the Verden garden of medicinal plants and the "Garden in Accordance with the *Capitulare de Villis*" of the Oerlinghausen Archeological Open Air Museum, where you can immerse all your senses in the ancient world of herbal medicine.

and pilgrims brought from distant regions. The range of healing plants recorded in the Plan of St. Gall—an intricately detailed 9th-century architectural drawing of the monastic island of Reichenau on Lake Constance—served as a model for many a cottage garden in Europe for centuries to come.

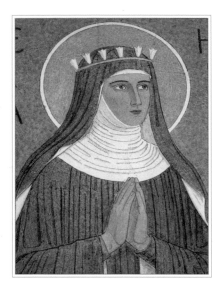

Hildegard of Bingen

Hildegard of Bingen (1098–1179) was one of the most famous healers of her time. First a nun in the Benedictine order, then the abbess of Rupertsberg Monastery on the Nahe River, she was also a visionary, a poet and a composer. Heavily involved in politics, she advised both Friedrich Barbarossa (Frederick I, the Holy Roman Emperor) and Pope Alexander III. Hildegard founded two monasteries, and, thanks to her progressive writings, was venerated as a saint during her lifetime.

Many followers of natural medicine regard the therapeutic methods of this Benedictine abbess as the origins of modern herbal medicine, because Hildegard managed to "marry" folk knowledge with the medical traditions of Greece and Rome. She used not only common, mostly Mediterranean herbs and exotic spices, but also native European plants, such as wild thyme, marigold and nettle. She was also the first person to use the vernacular plant names as well as the Latin names in her writings.

The Late Middle Ages and the Start of the Modern Era

Over the centuries, knowledge about the uses and benefits of medicinal herbs was recorded in an increasingly systematic manner. In the late Middle Ages, this knowledge was included in the curriculum of medical schools. At the same time, patient care increasingly shifted away from the monasteries and into the hands of secular physicians. Three cities became the most important centers for the academic study of medicine: the small southern French town of Montpellier; the ancient Italian city of Padua, situated west of Venice; and, a little later, Paris.

The *Circa Instans,* probably the most important medieval work on medicinal herbs, was published in the middle of the 12th century in the Italian town of Salerno. It was likely authored by a member of the famous Platearii family of physicians. It comprised some 270 plant portraits, which detailed not only each plant's range of effects but also its specific areas of application, and included possible substitutes. The book was quickly distributed across Europe and, together with other standard reference works, formed the basis of the great encyclopedias of the early modern age.

But certain standards needed to be developed in order to guarantee the quality and efficacy of drugs. Thus, in 1498, the first pharmacopoeia (book of medicines) was published. Initially, only pharmacists in the city of Florence had to abide by its rules, but within 50 years, pharmacists in many other areas of Europe had followed suit.

Meanwhile, Christian churches fought vehemently against the secularization of medical knowledge and the popularity of folk medicine. Witch hunts and the Inquisition claimed thousands of lives. Many of the victims were women, accused of being witches and heretics because, among other reasons, their age-old natural remedies often brought relief in cases where the church and male-dominated medicine had failed. As the Christian church expanded, numerous "pagan" medicinal herbs had been given Christian names; for example, St. John's wort (formerly known as goatweed, chase-devil or Klamath weed) and St. George's herb (valerian or all-heal).

A Second Heyday

During the Baroque Period, herbal medicine flourished once more. Books on herbs—often comprehensively illustrated— were written not only for physicians but also for educated and wealthy laypeople. Worthy of particular mention is the herb book by Eucharius Rösslin the Younger. This book was initially published in Frankfurt in 1533 and was revised and expanded several times; the final edition appeared in 1783. Rösslin's book helped preserve the knowledge of monastic medicine into the early 19th century, thus laying the foundation for "popular medicine" as it is still practiced today.

Carolus Linnaeus (1707–1778), who is also known by the names Carl von Linné or Carl Linnaeus, succeeded to an even greater degree than the academics of Renaissance Florence in the systematic cataloging of the plant world. Indeed, the great Swedish naturalist created the modern classification system known as "binomial nomenclature"; that is, the classification of living things according to genus and species names. It is still regarded as the standard scientific reference work today—across the entire world.

During the course of the Counter-Reformation in the 16th century, monastic medicine had regained some of its importance. Many of the newly founded monasteries had pharmacies that supplied both established physicians and laypeople with medicines. This state of affairs remained unchanged until the beginning of the 19th century, when many church estates were expropriated as a result of secularization movements.

Novel Drugs Conquer the World

The decline of the monasteries was only one of the reasons herbal medicine gradually lost its importance during the 19th century. As scientific methods advanced, physicians and pharmacists were more frequently able to isolate the active substances in medicinal plants, such as the morphine in opium, the strychnine in nux vomica, the quinine in cinchona, and the acetylsalicylic acid (the main ingredient in Aspirin) in willow bark.

The ability to manufacture these pure active components opened up an entirely new branch of medicine: the pharmaceutical industry. The manufactured medicines were a success—and not only in financial terms. At last, the quality of a remedy could be guaranteed. And because it would always meet the same standard, it became possible to create authoritative instructions for dosages. An additional benefit was that these isolated substances often worked faster than the "complete" plant.

This did not spell the total demise of natural medicine, as is often assumed.

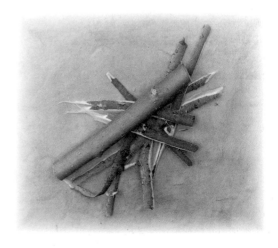

For many decades, much of the population continued to prefer natural treatments. However, healing plants played an increasingly minor role. Instead, improvements in health were sought from other natural elements, such as light, air, warmth, water and exercise. The Bavarian priest Sebastian Kneipp (1821–1897) was one of only a few exceptions. Kneipp regarded medicinal herbs as one of the five bases underpinning his holistic natural therapies. He believed herbs assisted in the prevention and treatment of diseases and that they should be administered internally as tisanes (teas) or juices; applied externally in the form of ointments or oils; or added to compresses, poultices and baths.

It would take nearly another 100 years, until the middle of the 20th century, before scientists started to seriously investigate medicinal herbs. Sales of herbs continue to rise today. According to recent statistics, tons of medicinal herbs are imported to Europe every year. And it's not only exotic plants, such as ginseng, that are in demand; indigenous herbs are, too, to make highly desirable oils and ointments.

The Return of the Natural Pharmacy

In the first few decades of the 20th century, there was widespread euphoria and certitude that everything could be produced synthetically, thereby "improving" on nature. However, a damper was put on these hopes in the latter part of the century. People increasingly realized that, along with the benefits of synthetic drugs, there came some definite drawbacks. This is why modern herbal medicine (known under the technical term *phytotherapy)* increasingly prepares drugs from plant extracts, backed by scientific research. The extracts are used to prevent and treat mild to moderately serious diseases.

Phytotherapy is excellent for self-medication, especially when used as a preventive treatment. In the case of more serious illness, plant-based medicines can be taken (preferably after a consultation with your physician) to effectively support conventional therapies; in some cases, they may even completely replace synthetic drugs.

Phytopharmaceuticals (the technical term for plant-based medicines) are manufactured on an industrial scale, and therefore contain active ingredients in reliable concentrations. During production, the plants or certain plant parts are chopped and pulverized, or their active ingredients are extracted. To ensure the quality of these products, only plants that have been certified and declared "non-harmful" may be used, and strict tests and quality standards are applied in order to guarantee the highest possible degree of safety. The efficacy and potential side effects of herbal medicines are also analyzed in detail.

On March 31, 2004, the European Union (EU) adopted a directive on herbal medicines, which came into force in 2011, after a transitional period of seven years. Since May of that year, only approved or registered traditional herbal medicinal products have been available in the EU. These are all categorized as safe and are labeled "traditional herbal medicinal product" or "administered in the traditional way."

Focus on Medicinal Plants

In recent years, medicinal plants themselves have increasingly become the focus of scientific inquiry. Unlike synthetically manufactured drugs, which contain a single, isolated active ingredient, a plant comprises a complex mixture of pharmacologically active substances. These are finely tuned to each other and in perfect balance. It is just like in nutrition: Even if a vitamin supplement contains a multitude of vitamins, it can never supply the body with as balanced a mix of vital substances as fresh fruits or vegetables can. Each plant is more valuable than the sum of its constituent parts—and this is why fresh food will always be more valuable to our health than artificial nutritional supplements. The same can be said for medicinal plants. Scientists around the world are researching these plants' active ingredients; that is, the components produced and stored by medicinal herbs. Only a fraction of these has been identified so far. What we do know, however, is this: It is the interplay of these substances that is responsible for each plant's efficacy.

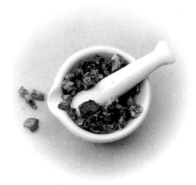

Important Plant Components

The most important, characteristic groups of substances in medicinal plants are the following.

- **Alkaloids:** These are nitrogenous substances produced by a plant (to protect it from predators, for example), which have a direct effect on the messenger substances in the human nervous system. While most alkaloids are poisonous substances, they can nevertheless act as a remedy if the correct dose is given. Their effects are many and varied—from stimulating (such as the caffeine in coffee, tea and cocoa) to numbing (such as the opium/morphine in poppies).

- **Bitter substances:** Bitter-tasting substances are contained, for example, in gentian, sage and wormwood. They stimulate the production of saliva, gastric juices and bile. They generally aid digestion, and are therefore components in numerous digestifs, or digestive bitters (you'll find my Bitters recipe on page 146).

- **Cardiac glycosides:** These active ingredients protect plants from being eaten, but they also affect the force and frequency of the human heartbeat. Probably the best-known example is the foxglove (digitalis) plant. But please, never, ever try it on your own!

- **Essential oils:** These volatile substances give each plant its individual, characteristic scent. In phytotherapy, they can be administered internally or externally for many different complaints. Essential oils can be pharmacologically active; for example, one might have an antiviral effect, such as tea tree oil, or a psychological effect, such as lavender (see more on aromatherapy on page 28).

- **Flavonoids:** These pigments (from the Latin *flavus*, for "yellow") are contained in a plant's cell sap. They often have an anti-inflammatory effect and are able to bind to free radicals, the highly reactive, aggressive oxygen molecules that cause cell damage. Among the most widely occurring secondary plant components, flavonoids are a plant's defense system, protecting it from attack by fungi, insects and other assailants. Flavonoids are abundant in marigolds, black cohosh and many other plants.

- **Mucins:** Mucus cannot be digested, so the protective layer it forms on the stomach wall cushions the organ from the aggressive effect of stomach acids. Plant mucins help create this type of protective

What are Drugs?

Drugs is not just the term for illegal narcotics. The word is also used to describe legal medicinal treatments, including medicinal herbs (or parts of them) that have been preserved through drying. (The term also applies to animals, microorganisms and resins that are used in the manufacture of medicines.) The English word *drug* might have come from the Middle Dutch term *droge vate*, which means "dry vats," referring to the contents of dry goods barrels. Among the herbal drugs, we distinguish between leaf, blossom, fruit, herb, rhizome, bark, seed and root drugs. As medicinal herbs mostly contain several medically active ingredients, they are often better tolerated by the body than synthetic drugs.

Let us turn to the example of Aspirin. Although this drug works faster than willow-bark tea (which would also have to be brewed first), this advantage is ultimately to the detriment of the stomach lining, as the active ingredient, acetylsalicylic acid, is rather aggressive. Aspirin also thins the blood, and this can lead to bleeding in the stomach. In the long term, a patient who uses Aspirin repeatedly may develop a gastric ulcer. However, these side effects do not develop with the natural treatment. In addition to acetylsalicylic acid, willow bark contains components that protect the stomach lining, and therefore the harmful side effects of the synthetic preparation are avoided. Medicinal plants often cause markedly fewer side effects than synthetic drugs.

layer; you'll find them in marshmallow root and psyllium (fleawort) seeds.

- **Pungent substances:** These "fiery" components—for example, the ones in fresh ginger—boost the production of saliva and gastric juices, and thus work miracles for morning sickness in pregnancy (see my pregnancy-friendly recipe for Ginger Candy on page 112). Administered externally, pungent substances stimulate the skin's pain and temperature receptors.
- **Saponins:** Combined with water, these components form a soap-like foam (the name comes from the Latin *sapo,* for "soap"). They have an expectorant and antibiotic effect, and stimulate digestion. Plants that are rich in saponins include ivy leaf and licorice root, which are used to combat colds and coughs.
- **Tannins:** Plants that contain tannins have an astringent (contracting), antibiotic and anti-inflammatory effect. They can bring relief in localized inflammatory diseases; for example, tannin-rich eyebright reduces eye inflammations (see my Eyebright

Compress recipe on page 46). Tannins may also help prevent cardiovascular diseases, joint complaints and other common symptoms of aging; try drinking Pomegranate Juice (page 137) to experience this effect.

Setting a New Trend

The back-to-nature movement has been able to gain ground not least because today's consumers are seriously interested in natural, gentle medical treatments. In 2010, a German survey on natural remedies showed that nearly 50% of people are convinced that these remedies work. They trust in nature's healing powers for a whole host of complaints, but especially for colds, gastric illnesses, insomnia, digestive problems and headaches. Accordingly, they increasingly use plant-based products to complement other treatments. (The eternal conflict between conventional and natural medicines seems to be resolved at last.) Last, but not least, there is a small bonus: Natural products are often less expensive than "normal" medicines—and sometimes they even cost nothing at all.

Health from Your Own Kitchen

People's growing interest in medicinal herbs is increasingly accompanied by their desire to make simple preparations at home. In some areas, our ancestors' knowledge has already regained a strong foothold, such as in the treatment of children's minor aches and pains. Increasing numbers of concerned parents are turning to eyebright drops for gummed-up eyes, or traditional onion bags if their offspring complain of painful ears (although my recipe for Parsley Poultice on page 36 is a more pleasant alternative). In fact, all age groups can benefit from nature's healing powers without too much effort. In the next few pages, you will learn about the easiest methods for creating natural remedies and their most popular applications. Then, in the large recipe section starting on page 33, you will find a suitable treatment for just about any health complaint.

Wild or Cultivated Plants?

Some of the medicinal plants required for the recipes in this book are cultivated on a large scale (for example, lavender). Others are still collected from where they grow naturally (for example, elder flowers). Herbs that are collected in the wild are usually of particularly high quality, because they are able to soak up lots of sunshine and energy, and grow untouched by human hands. However, if you want to collect medicinal herbs yourself, you'll need to be well versed in the world of plants. Some herbs have poisonous doubles, while others have protected status because demand for them is so high that wild stocks are steadily declining.

Whether you collect herbs yourself or buy them (or preparations made from them), keep the environment and species protection in mind. You can find out which plants are protected by contacting your local conservation authorities. Try to avoid using remedies that contain endangered plants, and ask your doctor or pharmacist for alternatives. If you are not certain of the status of a plant used in a specific remedy, contact the producer directly and ask whether they take note of species protection.

You can successfully grow many medicinal herbs at home: in your yard, on a terrace or balcony, or in a pot on a windowsill. When you pick herbs, their aromas will rise to your nose and have a first tentative effect on your body. If you want to preserve the riches of nature for the cold months, you can steep blossoms and herbs in oil or alcohol, or dry them gently in the fresh air or in the oven (at a maximum temperature of 175°F/80°C). Stored in an airtight container, in a cool place and protected from light exposure, they will keep over the winter.

To everyone who doesn't have time to dry home-grown herbs or wants to play it safe, I recommend buying medicinal herbs from the pharmacy. And always speak to your doctor to ensure the herbal remedies you're using are right for you.

Different countries have different standards for herbal medicines, however. In order to ensure that you're buying the highest-quality, safest products available, it's best to do your research and check the regulations where you live. In the United States, herbal medicines are not regulated the same way that conventional medications are, while in Canada, natural health products are evaluated and approved by the government. And in Europe, exacting standards for herbal medicines are adhered to, and high-quality herbal medicines are widely available.

The Most Common Forms of Natural Remedies

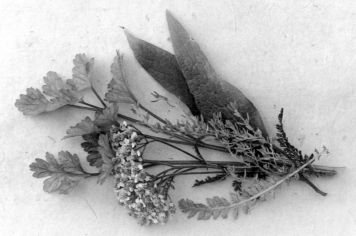

For generations, our ancestors simply used active ingredients directly from nature if they wanted to prevent a disease or treat its symptoms. They dried herbs for tisanes, mixed ointments, made macerations and infusions, or preserved the valuable components of medicinal herbs in other ways. Today, however, most of us rely on manufactured drugs, even though many people would actually prefer to combat ailments using natural remedies. Unfortunately, they no longer know how to make them.

Making Your Own Natural Remedies

In the following pages, you'll find out how to make use of the healing power of plants and how to produce your own remedies without too much effort. Starting on page 33, you'll find more than 60 recipes for remedies for a variety of complaints, and to use at every age and stage of life. I will explain each recipe to you, step by step. This will enable you to make a suitable remedy without any prior knowledge. And starting on page 153, I'll tell you which plants are particularly well suited for which ailments. In my selection, I didn't limit myself to plants that are local to me; I took full advantage of globalization and selected plants from far and wide for the natural pharmacy. Today, luckily, people are able to benefit from a cornucopia of highly effective medicinal plants from around the world, so you'll come across Ayurvedic, African and Chinese medicinal plants in this book. For many of the plants I profile, it has now been possible to prove scientifically why, how and on what they work. For other plants, this scientific proof is yet to come; for those, we can rely instead on the experiential knowledge built through (sometimes centuries of) traditional use.

Only the Best Quality Ingredients

Many of the remedies you'll learn about in this book are also available commercially—in varying degrees of quality. Some are excellent products. And while some readers may think that purchased remedies are always better than homemade because of legal requirements and controls, this is not always true. When you stand in your own kitchen, you decide what goes into a remedy. If you are using the purest essential oils and the freshest organic herbs, then you'll know for certain that this quality will be reflected in the final product. You won't have to trust someone else; you can know for sure.

Speedy Help from the Pharmacy

You won't always be able to have fresh herbs on hand when you need them. Therefore, it is helpful to know that there are a number of ways to obtain the active substances in medicinal plants if you're short on time or you lack the ingredients to make your own remedies. Below I summarize the most important drug forms. Ask your doctor or pharmacist which is best for you.

- **Pills:** Dried herbs are pulverized and then either pressed to make tablets or used to fill capsules. The advantage of this form is that you can accurately dispense a specific amount of an active substance and simply swallow the pills. For some herbs, which have peculiar flavors, such as greater celandine or bearberry leaves, tablets have the advantage of being neutral tasting (or at least they can be swallowed quickly).

- **Suppositories:** This dosage form is especially useful for children, who often don't like taking medicines. Adults may also, at times, benefit from using suppositories. These are inserted into the rectum or vagina, so in cases of intestinal disorders or vaginal mycoses (diseases caused by fungi), the active ingredients can quickly reach the place where they need to work.

- **Drops:** These are usually alcohol-based solutions of one or more herbs; alcohol-free versions are also available, especially for children (always check the label). In most cases, drops are taken orally. Drops are also a good solution when a plant's active substance is needed in a very small, defined area.

- **Syrups:** Thanks to their viscous consistency, syrups coat mucous membranes and directly supply them with the required active substances. They are, therefore, particularly well suited to the local treatment of throat and respiratory disorders.

Cautions for Natural Medicines

Unfortunately, it's a commonly held misconception that you can never go wrong with natural remedies. However, herbal remedies are also drugs and should therefore always be carefully prepared and dosed. Like conventional drugs, herbal remedies also contain active substances that may not be beneficial to the body in excessive quantities. In order to avoid habituation and any undesirable side effects, you should use neither proprietary remedies nor remedies prepared from the recipes in this book for a period of more than six weeks at a stretch. After this time, you should change to another medicinal herb that works in a similar way. If you're unsure, consult your doctor or pharmacist.

- **Rubs and ointments:** The active ingredients in an ointment are applied in a thin layer directly to the skin, where they can be immediately effective (for example, to treat dry skin or infected wounds). Rubs and ointments may also be applied to the skin in order to reach underlying organs, such as the bronchi, muscles or joints—as you will know from using chest rubs or rheumatism ointments.

- **Mouthwashes:** These remedies are usually diluted in water and are particularly well suited to treating mouth and throat inflammations. Gargling allows the active ingredients to reach even the farthest corners of the oral cavity.
- **Herbal teas or tisanes:** These drinks are made by pouring boiling water over dried plant particles and steeping them so that the active ingredients are released.

Teas

Brewing a tea from medicinal herbs is probably the easiest and quickest way to make use of nature's healing powers. Teas are especially successful at treating a general lack of well-being, as well as for minor complaints, such as gastrointestinal problems, colds, restlessness and nervousness. They have also proven their worth in treating acute inflammations of the bladder or kidneys, because they help flush out and detoxify the affected body parts at the same time. Yet, as gentle as teas may be, they, too, are natural remedies and are therefore not suitable for long-term use. As a rule, a single type of tea should not be drunk for more than six weeks at a time. Otherwise, the sustained use may lead to undesired side effects. These can vary considerably from case to case, and are dependent both on the individual's general constitution as well as the type of tea. Side effects may include headaches, nausea and stomach pains. After six weeks of drinking one type of tea, it is best to change to a different type with similar active substances.

Which Plant Parts Are Used?

Teas can be prepared from different parts of a plant. In some plants, most of the active components are concentrated in the leaves; in others, they are found in the flowers—or they may be in both parts. In still other plants, the roots or bark may be especially valuable. You can prepare a tea from either freshly picked or dried plant parts, and you can use a single herb or a mixture of different herbs—in the past, healing blends often included 20 or more different plants. In the case of blends, there is usually a main ingredient that most closely applies to a specific complaint. In tea blends, there can also be a variety of supportive ingredients, which are also beneficial for a particular ailment but play a lesser role. So-called accent or aromatic ingredients enhance the flavor and the presentation of the tea.

Cover Up

In my recipes, you'll probably notice that I repeatedly ask you to cover the pot or cup while the tea is steeping. There's a good reason for that. The essential oils, which contain all the actual goodness, easily evaporate along with the steam, dissolving into thin air just like that. If the tea is not covered as it steeps, it will taste the same but will no longer give you any benefits.

Fresh or Dried?

When you use fresh herb and plant material, always make sure that it has not been chemically treated. That's why it's best to use organic store-bought herbs or those from your own garden. If you collect herbs in the wild, make sure to pick them at some distance from roads with heavy traffic. These days, you can find dried herbs in every well-stocked supermarket, but it's better to buy them from an herbalist's shop, where the quality and the level of active substances in the herbs are guaranteed.

And speaking of levels of active substances: The best way to preserve them in herbs is through drying. Stored in an airtight container in a cool, dark place, dried medicinal plants will keep for about one year. The best storage options are dark glass containers or cans. Plastic containers are not as useful, because they can absorb some of the essential oils from the plants.

How Do I Make a Tea?

You may be saying to yourself, "I already know how to make tea!" And this is probably true for the most common method, infusion. Depending on the plant, however, other methods (maceration or decoction) may be used in order to obtain the maximum effect.

Infusions

The term *infusion* comes from the Latin *infundere,* meaning "to pour in." To make one, pour hot or boiling water over fresh or dried plant parts (leaves, flowers or chopped roots) in a teacup or teapot. Cover and let steep for about 10 minutes. Finally, strain the liquid and the tea is ready to drink.

If you want to drink multiple cups of an infusion over the course of a day, you can, of course, freshly prepare it each time. Alternatively, you may want to brew a large batch in the morning, then transfer the tea to an insulated teapot or Thermos.

Tea Tips

Many medicinal teas taste bitter. The good news is that you can sweeten them. Simply stir a small spoonful of honey into the tea, even if this is not explicitly mentioned in the recipe.

It is vitally important that you leave a tisane to cool to drinking temperature first. If it is too hot, many of the health-enhancing substances will be lost (for example, certain enzymes, vitamins and amino acids).

Tea connoisseurs may consider this an unforgivable sin. However, in healing tisanes, the health benefits are more important than the flavor.

Macerations

To make a maceration, or cold infusion, cover medicinal plants with cold water (instead of the boiling water used to make hot tea) and let steep for several hours or overnight. This method is mostly used for plants that contain heat-sensitive components, such as mucins; Fenugreek Extract (page 89) is a good example of this technique. After eight to 12 hours, the plant will have released all of its active substances into the water, and you'll only have to strain the liquid before using it. In fact, preparing a maceration is easy, if you don't mind the waiting time.

There is a minor disadvantage to this preparation method: Any germs present in the plant mixture will not be killed during the maceration process, as they would in a boiling-water infusion. If you want to play it safe, simply heat the cold infusion briefly after straining it. This will kill bacteria but will not affect the infusion's efficacy.

Decoctions

For tea ingredients that are hard, such as bark or roots, simply infusing them in boiling water won't release a sufficient level

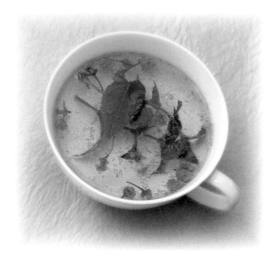

of the active substances. Therefore, place the plant parts in a saucepan of water and slowly bring the mixture to a boil. Simmer over low heat for 10 to 30 minutes. Strain the liquid through a fine-mesh sieve, and it's ready to use.

One advantage of making a decoction is that any germs present on the plant parts are reliably killed. However, some of the active substances can evaporate along with the steam, so always cover the saucepan with a lid to ensure the effectiveness of the finished decoction.

Tinctures

A tincture is an alcohol-based solution that contains the essential compounds of a plant. This type of preparation is recommended particularly when a healing plant contains active substances that are not water-soluble.

How Do I Make a Tincture?

A tincture is a little like a good wine: It needs to age. To make one, place the herbs in a large preserving jar and cover them completely with drinking alcohol (such as vodka, not the rubbing alcohol found at the pharmacy). And when I say "completely," I mean completely—any plant parts that are not covered by the liquid will go moldy. For the alcohol, you can use any clear spirit with an alcohol content of at least 38%. If the alcoholic strength is any lower, the mixture will not keep for very long.

Steep the alcohol and herb mixture in a warm place for two (or, better, four) weeks. Warmth encourages maturation. In summer, a south-facing windowsill is a good position; in winter try a place near a radiator. After this period of aging, strain the finished tincture through a fine-mesh sieve into a dark bottle. The dark part is extremely important! Exposure to light is desirable during the aging process, because it encourages the alcoholic extraction of the compounds in the herbs, but it significantly shortens the shelf life of a tincture.

In a dark bottle, a tincture will keep for a minimum of one year, often much longer. Even then, it does not "go bad" in the traditional sense, but its healing properties will slowly diminish.

Oil Infusions

Oil can be used in place of alcohol as a vehicle, or solvent, for extracting the active components of a plant. If you are planning to apply the finished oil infusion to your skin, use an oil with good skin-care properties, such as avocado or almond oil. Both oils contain many vitamins, and also rehydrate, tone and moisturize the skin. These oils add a cosmetic benefit to the effects of a plant's active components. These oils are, however, not cheap: a small, 8-oz (250 mL) bottle of good-quality cold-pressed avocado or almond oil will cost between $8 and $12.

If skin care is not your main concern, you can use a less expensive oil, such as sunflower oil. A not-too-pricey olive oil is also excellent as a base for oil infusions. Oils that contain polyunsaturated fats, such as evening primrose oil, are not suitable, because they perish too quickly.

How Do I Make an Oil Infusion?

To make an oil infusion, place the herbs in a preserving jar and cover them with slightly warmed oil (caution: again, the herbs need to be completely covered). Let the mixture steep in a warm place for two to four weeks. After that, strain it through a fine-mesh sieve. Stored in a cool, dark place, an oil infusion will keep for at least six months.

The Best Oils for Oil Infusions

- **Almond oil:** This oil moisturizes and soothes the skin. It is readily absorbed, very well tolerated and suitable for all skin types.
- **Apricot kernel oil:** This rich, nourishing oil contains many vitamins and boasts excellent skin-care properties. It firms the body's tissues and stimulates cell regeneration.
- **Avocado oil:** This very rich oil protects the skin from environmental ravages. However, it is not suitable for all skin types, nor for infants' skin.
- **Jojoba oil:** This is a good base oil for all skin types, and it has particularly nourishing characteristics.
- **Olive oil:** This extremely rich oil is particularly well-suited for use on dry skin.
- **Sunflower oil:** This oil has rehydrating, smoothing and anti-inflammatory properties.

Healing Vinegars

Another method of storing the active components of medicinal plants is to make vinegar extracts. This may sound complicated, but it isn't. All you do is pour good-quality vinegar (see below) over selected medicinal herbs and, in time, they will release their active substances into the liquid.

Vinegar is a veritable "miracle cure" in herbal medicine. One reason is that every cell in the body needs acetic acid (the acid that constitutes vinegar) to produce energy. In addition, it is much easier for the body to make use of the active substances in fruits, vegetables, and herbs when vinegar is involved.

Personally, I like to use organic apple cider vinegar as the base for my medicinal vinegars. It contains all the healthy properties of an apple, such as potassium, vitamins and pectin. In addition, apple cider vinegar also contains amino acids and enzymes that boost digestion, promote detoxification and support healthy intestinal flora. That is why it is my favorite among the vinegar varieties.

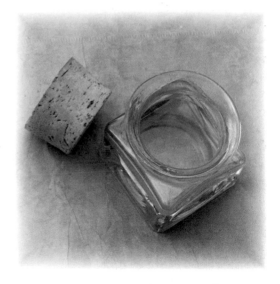

How Do I Make a Healing Vinegar?

Making a vinegar extract is very easy. As you would for an oil infusion (see above), place the herbs in a large preserving jar and cover with vinegar (again, ensuring that all of the plant parts are covered). Depending on the recipe, let the mixture steep for two to four weeks. When it's finished steeping, strain it through a fine-mesh sieve into a

Vinegar	Properties
Apple cider vinegar	Regulates blood pressure; lowers cholesterol levels; protects intestinal flora
Elderberry vinegar	Helps fight infections and inflammations
Fig vinegar	Mild laxative; improves concentration; slightly brightens mood
Honey vinegar	Mild enough that it agrees even with very sensitive people; has antibacterial properties; soothes mucous membranes
Pineapple vinegar	Eliminates water; has anti-inflammatory properties; promotes calcium absorption in bones
Red wine vinegar	Prevents arteriosclerosis; regulates cholesterol levels; improves digestion
Whey vinegar	Regulates intestinal flora; fights allergies; detoxifies
White wine vinegar	Fights inflammation, especially in urinary tract infections; generally said to have calming, uplifting effect

dark bottle. Stored in a cool, dark place, a healing vinegar will keep for several years.

How Do I Use It?

Healing vinegar can be used in many different ways. Here is a short list of common methods:

- **Internally (to boost intestinal activity):** Stir 1 tbsp (15 mL) healing vinegar into a generous ¾ cup (200 mL) water and drink in the morning, on an empty stomach.
- **As a bath additive:** Mix 1 cup (250 mL) healing vinegar into bathwater.
- **As a mouthwash (to detoxify the mucous membranes lining the mouth):** Stir 1 to 2 tbsp (15 to 30 mL) healing vinegar into a glass of water and swish around the mouth.
- **For gargling (to treat sore throats or tonsillitis):** Stir 2 tbsp (30 mL) healing vinegar into a glass of water and gargle.
- **In compresses:** Stir 1 tbsp (15 mL) healing vinegar into about 7 tbsp (100 mL) water, dip a clean cloth into the mixture and apply to the affected area for a short period of time.

Inhalations

Hot steam containing essential oils of medicinal plants will unblock a stuffy nose, moisturize irritated sinuses and soothe a cough. This is why inhalations have proven highly successful, especially for respiratory tract illnesses.

How Do I Make an Inhalation?

To prepare an inhalation, pour 4 to 8 cups (1 to 2 L) boiling water into a large bowl, then add six to 10 drops of an essential oil (see list, opposite page) or a generous ¾ cup (200 mL) of a tisane (for example, chamomile tea). On page 71 you'll find my recipe for a special oil blend that's ideal for inhalation.

To use the mixture, drape a towel over your head and hold your head directly above the rising steam. Make sure that the towel covers both your head and the bowl so that the beneficial steam cannot escape at the sides. The hot steam calms irritated sinuses as you breathe it in, and the essential oils that have been released will do the rest. Via the lungs, the healing substances also get into the bloodstream and can therefore become active throughout the body.

Careful, though: The steam is very hot! You'll automatically adjust your distance from the bowl until it is right for you, but there is still a danger of being scalded if the hot water sloshes out of the bowl, so place the bowl on a steady surface. Some essential oils, such as eucalyptus, may also irritate your eyes.

It's even safer to use an inhaler designed for this purpose, which you can find at a pharmacy or health care supply store. There are inexpensive plastic inhalers with shaped mouth- and nosepieces that seal firmly against the skin so that steam cannot escape. More complex devices may cost more than $150. It's very important that you clean the inhaler each time you use it. Let it dry completely so that no bacteria can grow in it. For some brands, you can clean the mouth- and nosepieces in the dishwasher.

How Long Do I Inhale For?

No matter which inhalation tools you choose to use, if you are ill you should ideally inhale two to three times a day for five to 10 minutes at a time. If inhaling makes you cough, the steam is probably too hot. However, the cough may also be a reaction to the added essential oils. If a little cold air or a swig of cold water do not

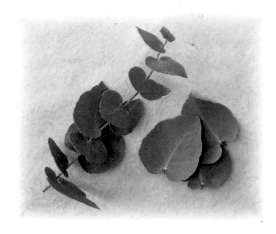

bring any relief, stop the inhalation and try a different mixture another time.

The Best Oils for Inhalations
- **Chamomile:** This plant is often used for coughs and sneezes, thanks to its strong anti-inflammatory powers. Chamomile inhalations are also very effective against acne.
- **Eucalyptus:** This herb has a mild laxative effect, improves concentration and slightly improves the mood.
- **Field mint:** Also known as wild mint, corn mint or Japanese mint, this is the base of a popular medicinal plant oil. It frees the air passages, fights headaches and soothes inflammation.
- **Niaouli:** This oil has antiseptic qualities, which means it acts as an expectorant. It is often used to treat rhinitis and sinusitis.
- **Spruce:** This oil unblocks the nose, and is particularly suitable for treating sinusitis.

Compresses and Poultices

A compress allows you to apply an herb's active substances directly to a specific area of the body via the skin. Even without any herbs, a compress promotes blood circulation and thus stimulates the body's self-healing powers. Active plant ingredients with medicinal properties increase and support this beneficial effect.

Compresses are very successful, particularly in the treatment of children. They perceive them as soothing, and they don't have to swallow any bitter medicines.

How Do I Make a Compress or Poultice?

A compress or poultice usually has three layers:

- **The inner cloth:** Soak a thin cotton or linen cloth (such as a tea towel or cotton handkerchief) in a tea, tincture or oil infusion. Or cover the cloth with balm or an extra-thin mash. For a poultice, place entire plant parts on the cloth, as in my Lemon Poultice (page 78). No matter what medicine it contains, place the inner cloth firmly, but not too tightly, on top of or around the affected body part, covering it completely.
- **The middle cloth:** A dry cloth forms the second layer. It has to be larger than the inner cloth and must cover it completely. A terry-cloth towel is the best choice.
- **The outer cloth:** Finally, the inner and middle cloths are covered with an even thicker layer. The best choice is a blanket or a thick cotton cloth; for leg (calf) compresses, a pair of thick woolly knee-high socks is ideal. Compresses applied to the ears can be held in place by a headband.

Some compresses consist of only two layers, such as the Lemon Poultice mentioned above, which is used to treat a sore throat. The throat is sensitive to constriction, so we generally use only two layers (the inner and middle cloths described above) over it.

Compresses (Hot and Cold)

You can use compresses for all sorts of purposes and to treat a variety of different ailments:

- Hot compresses relax body tissues. They may stay in place for up to 90 minutes. Well-known examples are chest compresses and liver compresses.
- Cold compresses, such as pulse or throat compresses, reduce swelling and boost the skin's eliminatory function, thus helping to soothe pain. They are removed (or replaced) after five to 15 minutes (that is, as soon as they start warming up).

Whether you're using a hot or cold compress, once you have taken it off, you should continue to rest on the couch or bed for a while. Do so for exactly the same length of time that the compress was applied.

Type of Compress	Used to Treat	Proven Remedy to Add
Chest	Cough, bronchitis, pneumonia	Lavender
Throat	Sore throat, hoarseness	Apple cider vinegar
Liver	Liver problems, often in conjunction with dietary changes; stimulates liver function; promotes detoxification	Yarrow
Pulse	Fevers, headaches; pulse compresses slowly lower body temperature and are suitable even for infants. Caution: Don't use on cold hands!	Lukewarm water
Back	Mucus buildup, by loosening viscous mucus in the bronchi; reduces muscle tension	Thyme
Leg	Fevers. Caution: Don't use on cold feet!	Apple cider vinegar

Herbal Baths

Bath Additive	Type of Bath
Spruce needles or rosemary	Stimulating energy bath
Lavender	Anti-stress bath
Neroli oil	Goodnight bath
Roman chamomile	Dry, sensitive skin treatment bath
Vanilla	Good mood bath
Vanilla and linaloe oil (2 drops of each)	Children's bath, particularly gentle on skin
Ylang-ylang	Fragrant bath

If you want to do something good for your body and use the skin as a medium to deliver helpful plant compounds, take a medicinal herb bath. All you have to do is jump in and enjoy.

How Do I Make an Herbal Bath?

One way is to "flavor" bathwater with a tisane made from medicinal herbs. To do so, place 0.35 oz (10 g) of medicinal herbs in a teapot and pour 2 cups (500 mL) boiling water over top. Cover and let steep for 10 minutes. Strain the tea through a fine-mesh sieve and add it to the bathwater.

Alternatively, you can put the medicinal herbs in a small linen bag, or even an old pair of tights. Tie tightly to close and hang this "teabag" directly in the bathwater (it's best to tie it to the faucet so that it hangs under the spout). Squeeze the bag from time to time to release the active substances in the herbs.

Using Essential Oils for Herbal Baths

Another method for making an herbal bath is to enrich the bathwater with the essential oils of a medicinal herb. Depending on the type of plant and the desired intensity, between four and 10 drops of essential oil are added to the tub. As you know, oil and water do not blend, so if you add the valuable essential oils directly, they will simply float on the surface of the water. To avoid this, you'll need to add a so-called emulsifier to blend the two liquids. Simply add 2 to 3 tbsp (30 to 45 mL) cream to the bathwater—it will create the desired emulsion of oil and water, plus it is good for your skin and makes it wonderfully soft. Full-fat milk and liquid honey are equally suitable emulsifiers. Oh, and yes, you can simply combine the essential oils with the cream, milk or honey in a cup in the kitchen, and then add the fragrant mixture to the hot bathwater.

How Long Do I Spend in the Tub?

How long you stay and at what temperature you wish to relax in the tub are entirely up to you. The guideline is to stay in the bath for at least 10 minutes so that your body can absorb enough of the active substances in the herbs. The water temperature should be roughly in line with your body temperature (95°F to 100°F/35°C to 38°C). Overly hot bathwater puts an unnecessary strain on the body's circulation and dehydrates the skin. On the other hand, you can't relax fully if the bathwater is too cool. One important note: Don't add any other bath products, such as bubble bath. These can noticeably reduce the effect of the medicinal herbs.

Aromatherapy

The point of aromatherapy is not simply to breathe in an active substance. Rather, the intense fragrance affects body processes; for example, it may stimulate hormone production. Scents arrive without detour directly at the diencephalon, or interbrain, where they affect the limbic system, which is thought to be the site of feelings and emotions in the brain. Once you know this, it is hardly surprising that certain scents improve mood, reduce anxiety or help people sleep better.

The body is also able to absorb essential oils via the skin (for example, in the form of an herbal bath; see page 27). Because these oils are fat-soluble, their active substances penetrate cell walls and travel through the bloodstream deep inside the body.

What Is Aromatherapy Oil?

An aromatherapy oil is the essence of a plant, which has been extracted, with the help of steam, from all or a part (such as the flowers) of a plant. Each oil has a characteristic aroma, and is also known as essential oil.

How Do I Recognize Quality?

Only use products that are labeled "100% pure essential oil." Don't use oils labeled "fragrance oil" or "nature-identical," which is simply another term for "synthetic." If the oil has been diluted, which may occasionally be the case for very expensive oils (such as iris essential oil), it is important to check which oil was used to dilute it. The higher the grade of the diluting oil, the better the result. St. John's wort essential oil, for example, is often blended with jojoba or almond oil because these oils offer excellent skin-care benefits. On the label of a high-quality essential oil, you'll find both the English and the Latin name of the plant. Labels may also include the term "G&A," which stands for "genuine and authentic," indicating a pure, unadulterated oil.

How Long Do Essential Oils Keep?

As a rule, you can keep essential oils for a year without any loss of quality if they are stored in a cool, dry, dark place. (Don't keep them in the fridge.) Flower oils, such as rose or lavender, can be kept for three years or even longer. If you're in doubt, simply smell the oil. If its scent or consistency has changed, that's a sign that the oil has "turned."

My Favorite Oils for All Situations

I recommend the following scents depending on the feeling or effect you wish to achieve.

- **Stimulating/invigorating:** Bergamot, grapefruit, mandarin or lemon
- **Relaxing/calming:** Anise, jasmine or lavender
- **Aphrodisiac:** Rose, vanilla or ylang-ylang
- **Concentration-boosting:** Lemongrass, lemon or cypress
- **Headache-busting:** Peppermint

Patch Test for Allergies

If you are concerned that you might be allergic to an essential oil, it is imperative that you test it before use. To do so, dilute the essential oil with a vegetable oil (for example, sunflower oil) at a ratio of 1:10—one part essential oil to 10 parts vegetable oil. Rub this mixture into the crook of your elbow and wait for 24 hours. If any skin irritation appears, you should not use this essential oil.

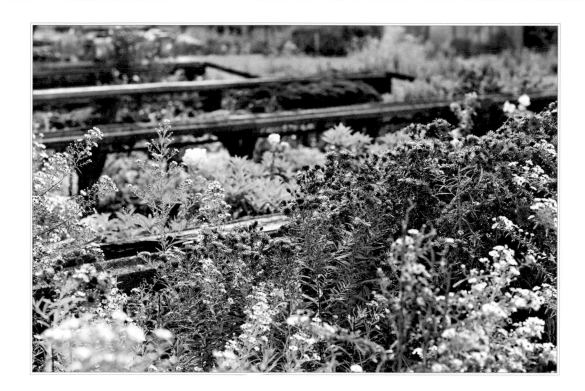

The Most Important Utensils

You should always have the following utensils on hand when you are working in your natural pharmacy.

Saucepans and Bowls

Small saucepans are great for heating or reducing liquids. If something needs to be heated in a water bath (that is, using a bain-marie, or double-boiler), the saucepan should be a little larger to make it easier to use.

Bowls can be of different sizes and may be made from metal, ceramic or plastic. Note, however, that the latter may take on the color of the contents. This is just a visual effect, so if it doesn't bother you, don't worry about it.

Mortar and Pestle

A mortar and pestle are a must for crushing seeds to release their essential oils. Mortars may be ceramic or earthenware. Personally, I recommend earthenware mortars. They weigh a lot more but they last forever, and they make grinding and crushing easy.

Bottles and Jars

Depending on which recipe you choose, you'll need a large or small bottle, a bottle with an eyedropper in the lid, a lidded cream or balm jar, or other types of storage containers. Among the resources listed on page 246, you'll find addresses of businesses from which you can easily purchase these various containers.

To make macerations, tinctures, oil infusions or healing vinegars, it's best to use clear glass preserving jars that can be tightly sealed. When the remedy is ready to be decanted, you should have a dark glass bottle ready for that purpose. Tinted bottles ensure that the remedy will stay protected from light and guarantees a longer shelf life (see page 22) for the mixture.

Funnel

When you've let a tincture steep for a week, then it runs down your hands as you decant it and trickles down the drain, you'll definitely wish you had bought a funnel. To avoid such frustrating pouring disasters, invest in this inexpensive tool from the start. Whether you decide to opt for a glass or a plastic funnel is purely a matter of preference.

Sieves

Fine-mesh sieves or tea strainers made from metal, cotton or plastic are widely available and perfect for straining mixtures. If very tiny particles need to be filtered out, you can use a coffee filter or a paper filter bag.

Gauze Cloths and Compresses

For some external treatments, you'll need a cotton cloth (such as a thin tea towel or a clean cotton diaper) or a gauze compress you can buy at the pharmacy. The size of the cloth will depend on the area that needs to be covered.

Labels

Information on shelf life is really useful— but it only helps if you write down the date your remedy was made. So before you store a bottle or jar, label it with the date when the contents were created. You can try small colorful labels designed for preserving jars or pretty ones in an ornate, retro style. It doesn't matter what you choose as long as the labels will reliably stick to the containers. And if you frequently ask yourself what exactly all those dark bottles contain, write the name of the remedy on the label as well.

Ingredients

You can easily purchase most of the ingredients featured in the recipes in this book at the pharmacy, at a specialty herb

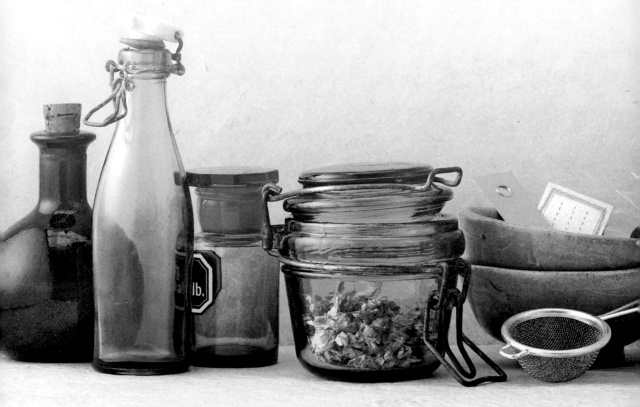

Reusing Bottles and Jars

If you'd like to reuse bottles and jars after a remedy is used up, rinse them thoroughly. Fill the container with boiling water, empty it and let it dry upside down on a clean towel before refilling it. If you don't refill jars and bottles immediately, rinse them again with boiling water to sterilize them just before filling. New containers should also be sterilized in this manner before their first use.

store or via the Internet. If you have no luck finding them, check the resources on page 246. Many well-stocked supermarkets also sell dried herbs—I advise you to opt for organic options whenever possible. I might be in danger of repeating myself too often, but the best part about creating homemade remedies is that you are totally in control of ingredient quality.

Anything Else?

Other items you'll need:

- **Digital scale:** For some herbal remedies, the weights of the ingredients are crucial to ensure the right proportions and ratios. If you're following the imperial measurements in the recipes in this book, a scale that weighs in increments of 0.01 oz is best for the small weights required for some of the recipes. If you're using metric measurements, your scale should weigh in increments of 1 g. In either case, a handy feature is a tare button, which allows you to place a container on the scale, then "zero" it so that it only weighs the contents.
- **Spoon:** You'll need a long-handled wooden or plastic spoon for stirring.
- **Teapot or teacup:** Models with built-in strainers are convenient; choose a teacup with a lid for best results.
- **Blender:** Either a countertop blender or a handheld (immersion) blender will work.

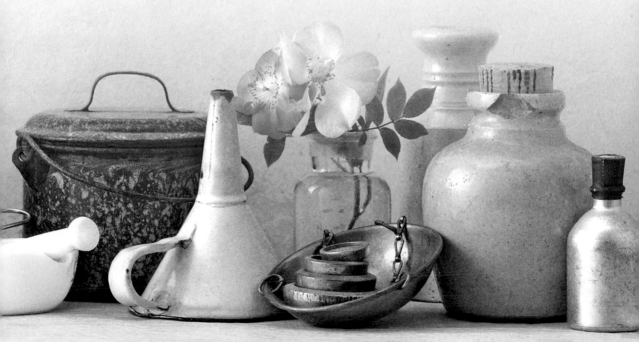

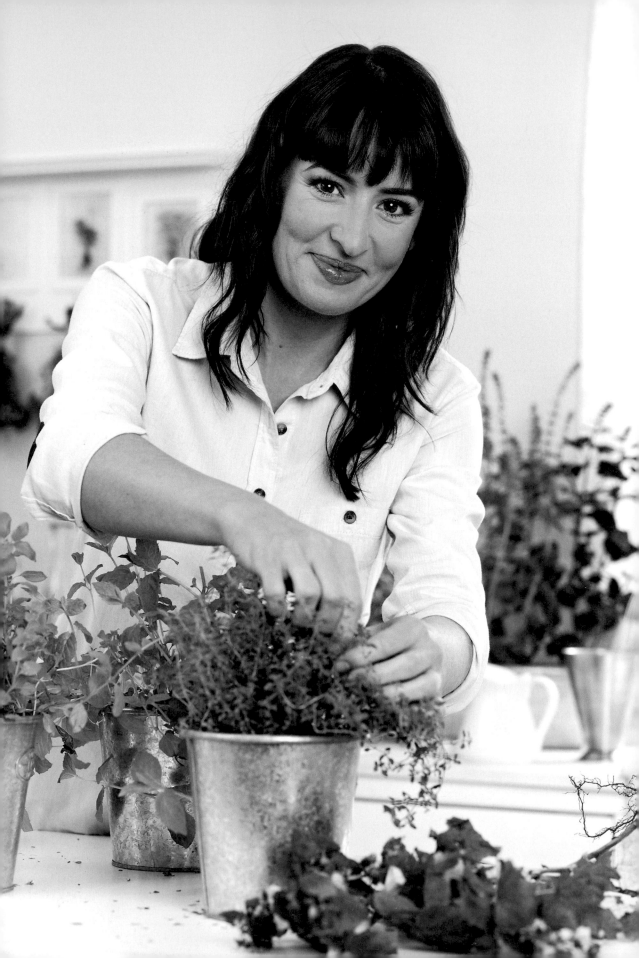

Recipes from Nature

Natural remedies do not need to come from the drugstore. You can easily make use of the healing power of medicinal plants at home and blend your own herbal teas, mix creams, or infuse oils and tinctures. To make it easy for you to start, I have gathered and written down my favorite recipes for every stage of life. Each of these remedies is perfectly easy to make. Simply try them out for yourself!

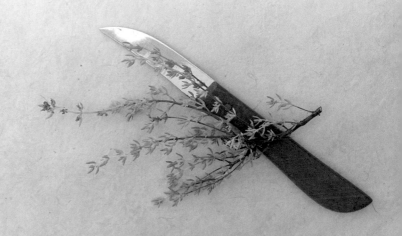

Remedies for Babies and Children

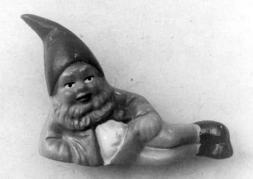

Medicines for children are always tricky. After all, you really want to be on the safe side here and take no risks. You want to help your little one without tormenting him or her, yet offer effective relief as quickly as possible. A sick child also poses a great emotional challenge to his or her parents.

Child-Oriented Medicine

In their search for gentle treatments, mothers and fathers have increasingly come across traditional methods. And it's true, especially for children, that natural medicine can often completely replace conventional cures. At the same time, natural remedies clearly have fewer side effects. No wonder then, that they are becoming more popular all the time.

Children are not just adults in miniature, however, and this is especially important in the natural pharmacy. Whether a recipe is suitable for children does not solely depend on its efficacy. If, for example, you give your child cough linctus (syrup) that tastes so disgusting that the child retches, you'll have a hard time standing your ground as "family doctor" in the future. Another example: Babies immediately taste bitter anti-colic drops in their milk; that means they'll resent Mom's medicine of choice for a long time to come. I've seen mothers weep,

spoon in hand, while begging their children, "Please, please, just open your mouth." You should not allow things to go this far.

What I am trying to say is that you have to start right away, in the early days of your child's life, to build his or her trust in Daddy as "medicine man" or Mommy as "medicine woman." With the recipes on the following pages, I want to help you create and sustain this level of trust. This is why, in my selection, I made absolutely certain to answer the following questions:

- What does the remedy contain?
- How does it work?
- What does it taste like?
- What does it feel like?
- How well is it tolerated?
- Have its benefits been proven?
- And, last but not least, how well do children accept it? That is, do children like taking this medicine?

My Favorite Recipes for Children

I have chosen the following recipes, created for the smallest people, with extra care. I've also added even more tips from my own practice than I did to the other recipes you'll find in this book, because life with children is always full of surprises. I've tried to indicate as wide a range of different remedies as possible. Here are the recipes you'll find in this chapter.

Parsley Poultice (page 36)

This is an alternative to the anti-inflammatory onion bags our grandmothers used to make. This is particularly good for children—it smells good, is quick to prepare and really very easy to use. Kids accept it readily.

Marjoram Ointment (page 37)

Rub a little of this remedy under your child's sniffly nose and the sneezing will soon stop.

Rose Gel (page 38)

This formulation is very effective against insect stings, minor burns and light sunburns. This efficacy is due not only to the active substances in the rose blossoms but also to the heavenly scent that helps the user quickly forget such minor ailments.

Anti-Colic Tea (page 40)

I recommend this tea to get rid of gas and colic during the first few months of a child's life. The herbs in it are anise, caraway, coriander and fennel; their active substances first relax a baby's tummy, then calm the entire child.

Clove Pack (page 41)

Cloves are the absolute best cure for toothaches. For the youngest children, a small pack they can bite down on is particularly helpful during teething.

Tormentil Tea (page 42)

The name of this herb sounds more like torment than relief, but it successfully and gently treats diarrhea, even in the youngest children.

Anti-Lice Shampoo (page 43)

Words you never want to hear: "Mommy, Jacob didn't come to school today; he has lice." If Jacob is your child's best friend, you can be fairly sure that your child will soon have a large number of these new, very loyal little friends, too. (Even if Jacob is in another class, there is still some risk.) In any case, this shampoo made with neem oil should prove effective at getting rid of the nasty little beasties.

Elderberry and Honey Syrup (page 44)

This tastes sweet and fruity, just the way you'd expect a cough syrup for children to taste. That means it won't be hard to make your kids swallow a spoonful of the remedy several times a day. Oh yes, I almost forgot: The recipe, of course, has the same beneficial effects on mommies and daddies with colds, too.

Eyebright Compress (page 46)

When the eyes are itchy or burn, or when they're already slightly gummed up, don't hesitate for too long. Just repeat the mantra, "Eyes closed, compress on." This compress will do exactly what you'd expect, soothing the irritation.

Heartsease Compress (page 47)

It may not be easy to guess what benefits wild pansies, or heartsease, might bring. Steeped in hot water, this herb has a beneficial effect that you would not expect from the name alone. It alleviates irritation and acts as an anti-inflammatory on skin.

Parsley Poultice

You probably know parsley from the kitchen rather than as a medicinal plant. But this herb is packed with vitamin C. It stimulates digestion and is often used to treat bladder and kidney infections. If it is applied externally, as in this poultice, it also has a strong anti-inflammatory effect.

When to Use It

For earache, discharge and infection of the middle ear.

How to Use It

The parsley poultice may stay on the ear for up to 2 hours. If the pain persists after application, make a new poultice and replace it on the ear.

Tip

You can also use an onion bag to fight an earache: Finely chop onions, place them on a cotton handkerchief and tie together. Children are usually not so keen on this remedy because of the strong onion smell.

You Will Need

- Sharp knife
- Cutting board
- Thin tea towel, gauze cloth or cotton diaper

| 2 | handfuls fresh flat-leaf or curly parsley sprigs | 2 |

How to Make It

1. Using a sharp knife and a cutting board, chop parsley (including stems) very finely. It should almost be a paste.

2. Spread the parsley paste down the center of a thin tea towel.

3. Fold the fabric over the parsley to make a pillow-shaped package. Place the poultice on the painful ear and hold it in place with a scarf or, even better, a woolly hat.

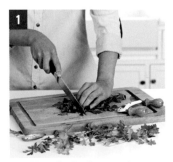
Very finely chop parsley.

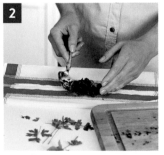
Spread paste on cloth.

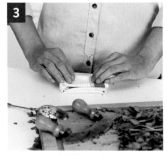
Fold like a pillow.

Marjoram Ointment

Marjoram is antibacterial and antispasmodic. It gently reduces swelling of the sinuses and makes breathing easier, without drying out the nose. Used internally, marjoram aids digestion and helps fight flatulence and abdominal spasms.

When to Use It

For head colds.

How to Use It

Rub a pea-size portion of the ointment just below and inside the nose.

Shelf Life

The ointment will keep for up to 2 months in the fridge.

Tips

Make sure to buy your marjoram from a pharmacy or an herbalist to ensure quality.

If your baby suffers from gas, massage his or her tummy in a clockwise direction with a little marjoram ointment.

You Will Need

- Mortar and pestle
- Glass measuring cup
- Large saucepan
- Spoon
- Fine-mesh sieve
- Lidded jar

1 tbsp	dried marjoram	15 mL
1 tbsp	butter	15 mL

How to Make It

1. Using a mortar and pestle, grind dried marjoram until it is a fine powder.
2. In a glass measuring cup set in a large saucepan of boiling water, melt butter. Using a spoon, stir in marjoram until well combined.
3. Using a fine-mesh sieve, strain marjoram mixture into a lidded jar. Let cool (mixture will harden).

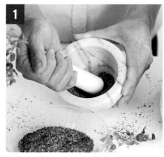
Grind marjoram using mortar and pestle.

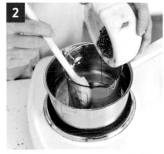
Stir marjoram into melted butter.

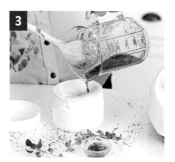
Strain into jar.

Rose Gel

The queen of flowers, the rose does so much more than merely look pretty. The flower has been highly valued for its scent and healing powers since the Middle Ages. People even seem to react to the scent of roses while they're asleep—a study has shown that it brings them pleasant dreams.

When to Use It

For insect stings and sunburns.

How to Use It

Apply a thin layer of the gel to insect stings or sunburned skin. It is wonderfully cooling and quickly brings relief.

Shelf Life

The gel will keep for 6 months in the fridge.

You Will Need

- Large glass measuring cup or wide-mouthed glass
- Small whisk
- Lidded jar

5½ tbsp	rose water (see tips, below)	80 mL
1¾ tsp	90% isopropyl rubbing alcohol	8 mL
1 tsp	powdered gelling agent (see tips, below)	5 mL

How to Make It

1. Pour rose water and alcohol into a large glass measuring cup.
2. Carefully sprinkle gelling agent over top.
3. Using a small whisk, stir mixture until gelling agent is completely dissolved. (This may take a few minutes; don't give up.)
4. Pour the gel into a lidded jar. Spread a thin layer over stings or sunburned skin.

Tips

Look for rose water in pharmacies or the specialty sections of supermarkets. You'll find a variety of powdered gelling agents at the drugstore or the organic food store, both from animal (gelatin) and vegetable (agar-agar) sources.

Exhausted moms (and others) may also use Rose Gel as an excellent firming and moisturizing facial mask. Apply the gel really thickly to your face, avoiding the areas around the eyes and lips. Leave it to work for 10 minutes, then wipe it off with a moistened cloth—finished!

For insect stings, a simple substitute for Rose Gel is apple cider vinegar. Drizzle it over stings to ease pain.

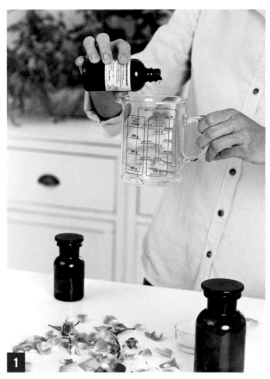

1. Combine rose water and alcohol.

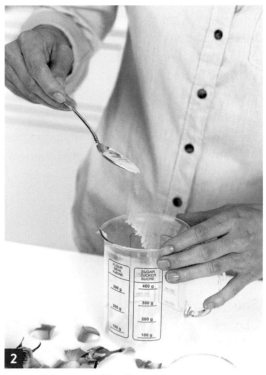

2. Add gelling agent.

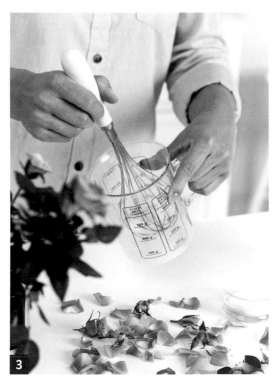

3. Stir well to combine.

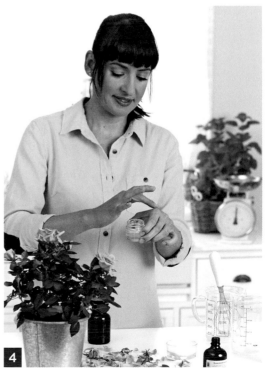

4. Thinly apply gel to affected skin.

Anti-Colic Tea

Anise, fennel, caraway and coriander are probably the most successful quartet in natural medicine for treating flatulence, stomach ache and bloating. They break up gases in the intestines the gentle way and quickly bring relief. This tea is exactly what little babies need.

When to Use It

For colic (also known as gripe).

How to Use It

Let your child drink the lukewarm tea, one small sip at a time.

Shelf Life

The tea blend will keep for at least 1 year.

Tip

Fennel tea from the drugstore or a specialty tea shop is a good substitute for this blend.

You Will Need

- Tea caddy
- Tea strainer
- Teacup

1 oz	aniseed	30 g
1 oz	fennel seeds	30 g
1 oz	caraway seeds	30 g
1 oz	coriander seeds	30 g

How to Make It

1. Spoon aniseed, and fennel, caraway and coriander seeds into a tea caddy. Shake to combine.
2. Place 1 tsp (5 mL) tea blend in a tea strainer inside a teacup.
3. Pour a generous ¾ cup (200 mL) boiling water over top. Cover and let steep for 10 minutes (if it's not covered, you will lose the valuable essential oils).

Caution

Your child shouldn't drink more than three cups of this tea per day—larger amounts can cause an overdose of the active substances.

This tea should not be drunk for more than 3 weeks in a row without a break.

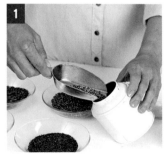
Combine seeds in tea caddy.

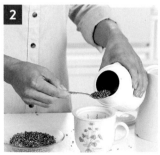
Measure tea blend into teacup.

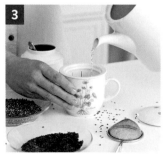
Pour boiling water over top.

Clove Pack

Cloves are not only an important spice for Christmas baking but also a tried-and-tested painkiller with a calming effect, particularly on teeth and gums. A clove pack is therefore particularly well suited as a "teething ring" if your child encounters problems when his or her first teeth appear. And it's quick to make, too.

When to Use It

For toothaches.

How to Use It

Gently chew and suck on clove pack. If you think the pack has been "sucked dry" (literally), simply replace it with a fresh one.

Tip

Some children cannot get used to the distinctive flavor of cloves. In that case, try violet root (found in pharmacies or organic grocery stores). Its effect is comparable but it has a more neutral taste, plus your child can chew on the root as is.

You Will Need

- Cotton handkerchief
- Strong ribbon or string

3 or 4   whole cloves   3 or 4

How to Make It

1. Count out the number of cloves preferred.
2. Place cloves in the middle of a cotton handkerchief.
3. Using a strong ribbon, tie securely to form a bundle. Let your child chew on the clove pack for as long as he or she likes.

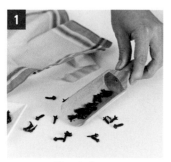
Count cloves.

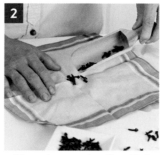
Place cloves on handkerchief.

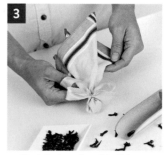
Tie into bundle with ribbon.

Tormentil Tea

Tormentil has had a firm place in natural medicine since the Middle Ages. Many benefits were ascribed to this plant—some even say it encourages a long life. The herb is very gentle yet effective for treating diarrhea, and therefore is suitable even for infants.

When to Use It

For diarrhea.

How to Use It

For an acute case, give your child up to two cups of tormentil tea during the course of a day.

Shelf Life

The dried root will easily keep for 1 year in an airtight container.

You Will Need

* Tea strainer
* Teacup

1 tsp	dried tormentil root	5 mL

How to Make It

1. Place tormentil root in a tea strainer inside a teacup.
2. Pour boiling water over top.
3. Cover and let steep for 10 minutes. Let cool slightly.

Caution

When infants suffer from diarrhea, they quickly dehydrate. If the affliction is severe or lasts for a long time, consult your physician right away in order to avoid any complications.

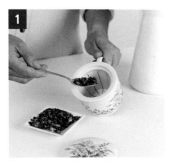
Spoon tormentil root into teacup.

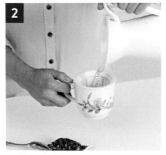
Pour boiling water over top.

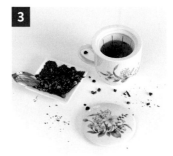
Let tea steep.

Anti-Lice Shampoo

Neem oil is extracted from the seeds of the neem tree. It has a pungent scent, but don't let that deter you. Lice have become resistant to many chemical anti-lice treatments, but the bothersome beasties have not yet managed to become immune to this herb.

When to Use It

For treating an attack of head lice and to prevent future attacks.

How to Use It

Wash your child's hair two or three times a week with this shampoo. Let it stand on the hair for about 10 minutes before rinsing. If lice have already made a home in your child's hair, carefully comb it with a lice comb, after washing but while still wet.

You Will Need

- Large glass measuring cup
- Shampoo bottle (8 oz/250 mL)

¾ cup + 2 tbsp	baby shampoo (or your favorite shampoo)	200 mL
1 tbsp	neem oil (see tips, below)	15 mL
2 tsp	neem leaf tincture	10 mL

How to Make It

1. In a large glass measuring cup, combine shampoo, neem oil and neem leaf tincture.

2. Pour mixture into a shampoo bottle.

3. Vigorously shake the bottle. The shampoo is ready to use.

Tips

If you just want to be good to your hair, simply add ½ tsp (2 mL) neem oil to your normal shampoo and shake well. It will give your hair body and sheen—and the oil will also prevent greasiness.

Look for neem oil and neem leaf tincture at the pharmacy. If you don't have time to make your own anti-lice shampoo, there are natural, herbal alternatives on the market.

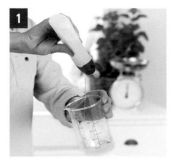

Combine shampoo, neem oil and neem leaf tincture.

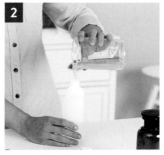

Transfer to bottle.

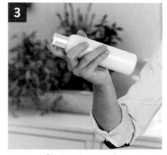

Shake vigorously.

Elderberry and Honey Syrup

Elderberry is known for its outstanding effectiveness in fighting colds and flus, and for strengthening the immune system. If the juice is sweetened with honey, even children will find it delicious.

When to Use It

For feverish illnesses.

How to Use It

At the start of a cold or fever, give your child 1 tsp (5 mL) of the syrup every 2 to 3 hours, letting it slowly dissolve in the mouth.

Shelf Life

Once opened, a jar will keep for about 6 months in the fridge.

You Will Need

- Saucepan
- Wooden spoon
- Preserving jar (2 cups/500 mL)

¾ cup + 2 tbsp	freshly pressed elderberry juice (see tips, below)	200 mL
10 oz	organic liquid honey	300 g

How to Make It

1. In a saucepan, heat elderberry juice, stirring with a wooden spoon.
2. Add honey and simmer over low heat, stirring, until reduced to moderately thick syrup, about 10 minutes.
3. Rinse a preserving jar with boiling water. Pour hot syrup into the jar and seal immediately. Let cool, then store the jar in the fridge.

Tips

Fever is not a disease in its own right but rather a symptom indicating that the immune system is trying to fight off an attack. It is a completely normal bodily reaction and initially nothing to worry about. You should, however, visit the doctor if your child is younger than three months old, if the fever lasts for more than three days without any obvious reasons, or if you're worried about your child's general condition.

Look for freshly pressed elderberry juice at natural foods stores or organic supermarkets.

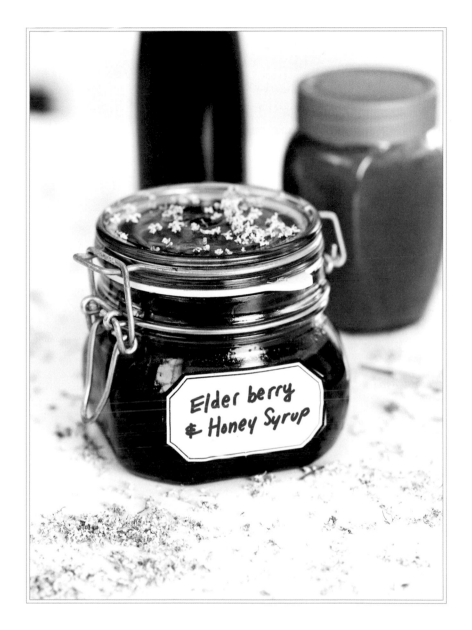

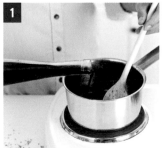

Heat elderberry juice.

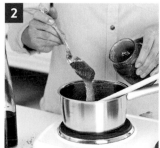

Stir in honey.

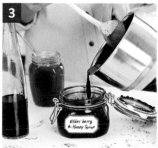

Pour into preserving jar.

Eyebright Compress

The name says it all! Eyebright is an effective herb for all eye diseases, and even young children can be treated with this remedy. The active substances in eyebright (glycosides, tannins and flavonoids) are antibacterial, anti-inflammatory and antispasmodic.

When to Use It

For inflammatory diseases of the eye.

How to Use It

Place the compress on the inflamed eye for about 5 minutes, or dab the affected eye several times a day with a fresh, moist compress.

Shelf Life

The tea will keep for 2 days in an airtight container in the fridge.

You Will Need

- Tea strainer
- Large teacup
- Gauze cloth or cotton pad

1 tsp	dried eyebright (or 2 tsp/10 mL fresh eyebright)	5 mL

How to Make It

1. Place eyebright in a tea strainer inside a large teacup.
2. Pour generous ¾ cup (200 mL) boiling water over top. Cover and let steep for 10 minutes. Let cool.
3. Dip a gauze cloth into tea. Lightly squeeze out liquid so that the compress is just moist, not wet.

Tips

Eye inflammations are usually infectious. Make sure, therefore, that you thoroughly wash your hands before and after touching the affected eye. Also make sure you use each compress only once.

If you want help fast, look for ready-made eyebright-based eye drops at the drugstore.

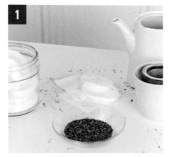
Place eyebright in tea strainer inside teacup.

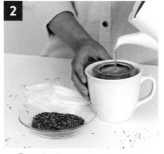
Pour boiling water over top.

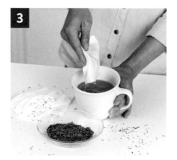
Dip compress into tea.

Heartsease Compress

The flavonoids and mucins contained in heartsease, or wild pansies, have a gently soothing, anti-inflammatory effect on the skin.

When to Use It

For rashes and itchy, inflamed skin, as well as to treat cradle cap.

How to Use It

You can apply the compress to the affected area several times a day. Remove it after 30 minutes or when your child no longer finds it soothing.

You Will Need

- Tea strainer
- Large teacup
- Teaspoon
- Gauze cloth or cotton pad

| 2 tsp | dried heartsease | 10 mL |

How to Make It

1. Place heartsease in a tea strainer inside a large teacup. Pour generous ¾ cup (200 mL) boiling water over top. Cover and let steep for 10 minutes.
2. Holding tea strainer over teacup, press heartsease with a teaspoon to remove liquid. Let cool.
3. Dip a gauze cloth into tea. Lightly squeeze out liquid so that the compress is just moist, not wet.

Caution

Skin compresses should only be handled by competent adults. This compress will provide relief, however, until you can get to the doctor or homeopath. It can also be used in combination with conventional treatments.

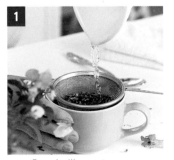

1 Pour boiling water over heartsease.

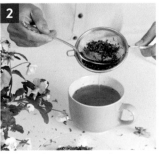

2 Press out liquid.

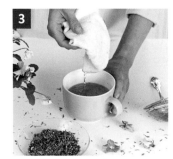

3 Dip compress into tea.

All Grown Up

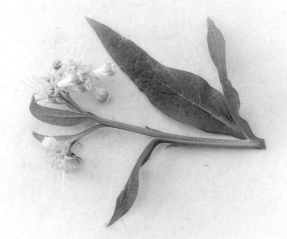

Small children, small problems. So, big children, big problems? Nonsense! The problems are just different. Accordingly, every parent's wish to treat complaints the natural way—quickly, gently and, above all, without side effects —is the same for big children as it is for little ones.

Of Prevention and Cure

Luckily, as they grow up, schoolchildren and teenagers become more understanding, and will (hopefully) accept medicines as a necessity. However, your offspring won't always cooperate as you might wish, and you'll have to expect some continued resistance. With older kids, there's often not an easy solution. But when younger kids are laid low, they'll usually give in—who wouldn't want to heal a sunburned nose or get rid of an annoying pimple as quickly as possible? This is your chance!

My Favorite Recipes for the Big Kids

In this chapter, you'll find effective recipes for typical health problems and ailments that affect children and young people between the start of school and puberty. In my experience, these remedies are all well accepted by kids.

Winner's Breakfast (page 50)
This truly is "food for thought," or at least food for brainpower and intelligence! A spoonful of flaxseed oil kick-starts intellectual power and is even said to have a positive, calming effect on children who suffer from hyperactivity. Sure, the kids will still have to knuckle down and do their homework. But this contribution from the natural pharmacy can help them recall what they've learned in a concentrated way during an exam. This recipe will warm up the gray matter and get it ready for learning.

St. John's Wort Oil (page 52)

Almost as bad as getting a kiss from Mom in front of their friends, the smell of (babyish) sunscreen is totally embarrassing for teenagers. And so, after a game of baseball or soccer, they might come home with a nose glowing red—and that turns typical teenage disdainful nose wrinkling into agony. This is a remedy to keep on hand for those who dare to get sunburned.

Comfrey Ointment (page 54)

Scuffles in the schoolyard, in the school gym or on the soccer field—you have to expect the odd sprain, bruise or pulled muscle. You, as your young savage's "family doctor," therefore, need plenty of pain-killing and swelling-reducing comfrey ointment in your natural pharmacy.

Bentonite Clay Face Mask (page 56)

Pimples are a normal part of puberty. They arrive because the production of sex hormones begins during those years, and it takes a while to establish the correct balance. For teenagers, however, pimples are a catastrophe. While it's not possible to totally banish these annoying companions, eating a vitamin-rich diet will help prevent other changes in the skin due to nutritional deficiencies. It will, at the same time, stimulate the healing process. The occasional meal of brown rice, wheat bran and lentils (full of vitamin B_5) is always a good idea. Pimples are, however, not all alike. Whereas some teens occasionally have a small one here or there, others hardly dare to leave home. Consult a dermatologist or homeopathic practitioner for serious cases of acne. For others, this mask will get rid of common puberty-related pimples.

Wound Cleanser (page 57)

Scuffles in the schoolyard, in the school gym or on the soccer field—oh, wait, I said that before! If these brawls result in the occasional open wound, however, simply applying an ointment won't do. First, the wound needs to be thoroughly cleansed, and this recipe is great for that.

Sage Candy (page 58)

Did I say that "big" children were more reasonable? Well, I meant during a relatively brief (sometimes hardly noticeable) period sometime between starting school and the onset of puberty. You can assume that, in midwinter, your 14-year-old will consider it absolutely out of the question to wear a scarf and hat, even if the temperatures have dropped to below freezing. You're therefore obliged to have some of these sore throat candies ready. These will suddenly seem cool when your child's voice eventually starts to crack.

Pine Rubbing Lotion (page 60)

It may sound old-fashioned, but this lotion is still the best remedy for sore muscles (and sports injuries). It's likely that the German soccer teams that won the World Cup in 1954 and 1974 (and perhaps even in 1990) rubbed their tired limbs with a lotion like this—so that should count for something with your cool teenager.

Spruce Bath Salts (page 62)

Do kids really get growing pains? Well, physicians are still not 100% certain about what causes some kids to get these tearing pains in the legs (usually in the knee joints and the calves), which occur mostly in the evenings. It is possible that they may be the result of ligament and tendon expansion. The occurrence and frequency of these pains differs from one child to another, but a relaxing bath with these salts will work wonders in any case.

Winner's Breakfast

Flaxseed oil strengthens the immune system and lowers cholesterol levels. Above all, its high content of omega-3 fatty acids (higher than in fish!) promotes concentration and memory. It is a true brain food, and it makes even the sleepiest kids alert and fit for everyday life at school.

When to Use It

For lack of concentration.

How to Use It

Enjoy this breakfast as soon as it's prepared.

Shelf Life

Flaxseed oil goes rancid quickly. Keep the oil in the fridge once the bottle has been opened, and use it up within 2 months.

You Will Need

- Cereal bowl
- Spoon

3.5 oz	seasonal fresh fruit (local, if possible)	100 g
3.5 oz	quark or strained cottage cheese (see tips, below)	100 g
1 to 3 tsp	cold-pressed organic flaxseed oil	5 to 15 mL
	Muesli or rolled oats (optional)	

How to Make It

1. Wash fruit. Cut into bite-size pieces, if needed, depending on what fruit you are using.

2. Spoon quark into a cereal bowl. Stir in flaxseed oil.

3. Stir in fruit, and muesli (if using).

4. Enjoy as a hearty, delicious breakfast.

Tips

Stir the flaxseed oil into the quark 1 tsp (5 mL) at a time. Flaxseed oil has a rather strong taste that is not everyone's cup of tea; your child's taste for it will determine how much you can add. It should be easy enough to sneak in at least one spoonful, however. If your child likes the flavor of the oil, you can happily add two or three more spoonfuls.

Quark is a traditional German fresh cheese. It is now available in some markets in North America. Strained cottage cheese or other fresh cheeses are fine substitutes. The percentage of milk fat in them is your choice.

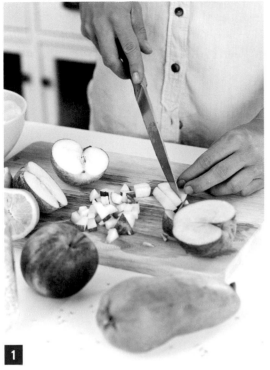

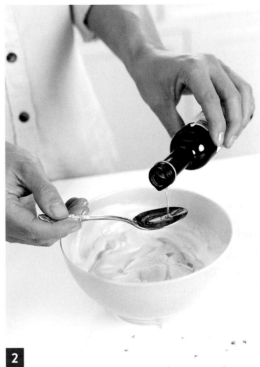

1 Cut up fruit.

2 Stir flaxseed oil into quark.

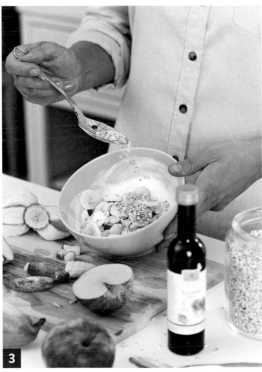

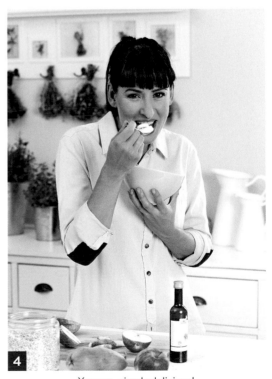

3 Stir in fruit, and muesli (if using).

4 Yummy—simply delicious!

St. John's Wort Oil

St. John's wort is one of the oldest and most analyzed medicinal herbs. You probably already know of the plant as a natural remedy for depression. But it is capable of much more: Used externally, it kills bacteria and stimulates healing. You can therefore make an excellent wound and massage oil from St. John's wort.

When to Use It

For burns, blunt trauma injuries, sunburns, aching joints and backaches.

How to Use It

Gently massage the oil into the skin over the affected area; use it as often as you like or until the pain disappears.

Shelf Life

This oil will keep for about 1 year in a cool, dark place.

You Will Need

- Preserving jar (2 cups/500 mL)
- Funnel
- Fine-mesh sieve
- Dark bottle

1	handful dried St. John's wort flowers and flower buds (or 2 handfuls fresh St. John's wort flowers)	1
	Good-quality organic vegetable oil (such as olive, almond or jojoba)	

How to Make It

1. Spoon St. John's wort flowers and buds into a preserving jar.

2. Pour about 10 times the volume of vegetable oil over top. All of the flowers need to be completely covered with oil. Place the jar in a sunny spot (a windowsill is best) for 6 weeks. Once a day, shake the jar vigorously like a cocktail shaker. After 6 weeks (yes, you need to be patient, but this shaking act is really easy), the oil will have turned blood red.

3. Using a funnel and a fine-mesh sieve, strain oil into a dark bottle. The flowers will have released all their active substances into the oil; they are no longer needed and can be thrown away.

Tips

You can use a second, clean preserving jar if you don't have a bottle to put the oil in.

There are ready-made equivalents of this oil. Check for it at drugstores and online.

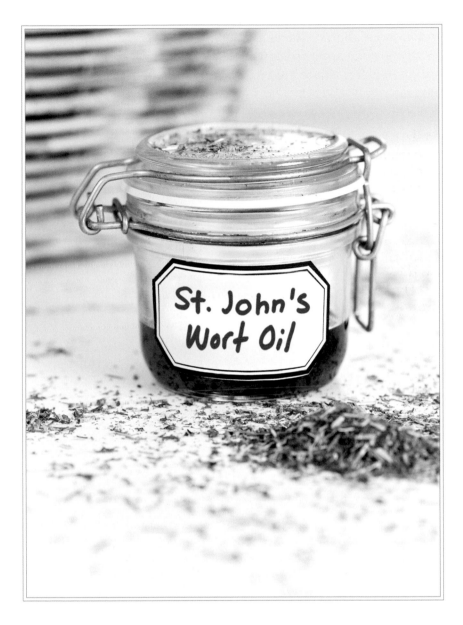

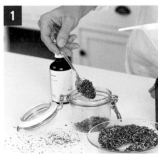

Spoon St. John's wort into preserving jar.

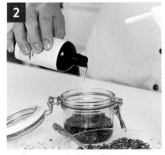

Pour vegetable oil over top.

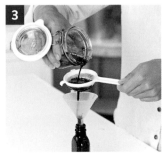

Strain finished oil into dark bottle.

Comfrey Ointment

Comfrey has anti-inflammatory, decongestant and analgesic properties. That's why many proprietary products are made with this medicinal herb. However, the only way to be absolutely sure that you are dealing with a pure, natural product is to prepare it yourself at home.

When to Use It

For bruises, strains, skin pinches and sprains, and to boost bone healing.

How to Use It

Apply the ointment to the skin over the affected area. Use it twice a day if possible.

Shelf Life

Comfrey ointment will keep for about 1 year in the fridge.

You Will Need

- Small saucepan
- Wooden spoon
- Fine-mesh sieve
- Large lidded jar or several small lidded jars

8 oz	Melkfett (see tips, below)	250 g
1	large piece fresh comfrey root, washed and cut in small pieces (or 3.5 oz/100 g dried comfrey root), see tips, below	1

How to Make It

1. In a small saucepan, carefully melt the Melkfett over low heat, stirring with a wooden spoon, without letting it sizzle.

2. Add comfrey root to melted Melkfett. Remove the pan from the heat. Let cool. Every day for 1 week, reheat mixture in a saucepan. (Don't let it boil.) As soon as the fat is warm, take the saucepan off the heat and let cool again.

3. On Day 7 (though it doesn't matter if you wait until Day 8 or Day 9), warm the mixture. Using a fine-mesh sieve, strain mixture into a lidded jar. Seal tightly.

4. Spread ointment over affected area.

Tips

Melkfett is a traditional German skin cream originally made to treat and protect cows' udders for milking. You can find it online and in some specialty stores.

Fresh comfrey root looks like it has just been pulled out of the dirt; this is why it needs a thorough washing under running water. But be gentle: The dark skin of the root needs to stay intact. (This step is not necessary if you are using dried root, which is usually sold already chopped.)

There are some good commercial comfrey ointments, and you can often find them for sale online.

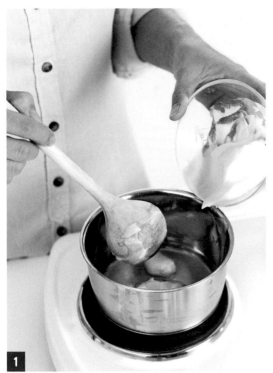

1

Melt Melkfett over low heat.

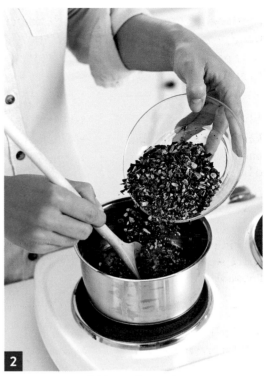

2

Stir in comfrey root.

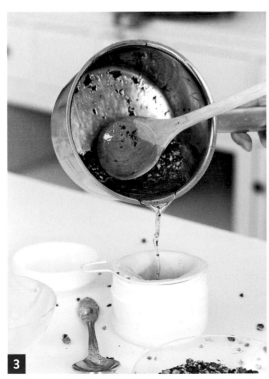

3

Strain mixture into lidded jar.

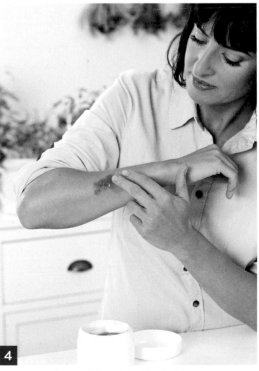

4

Apply ointment to affected area.

Bentonite Clay Face Mask

St. Hildegard of Bingen (see page 12) knew about the beneficial effects of bentonite clay back in her day, in the 12th century. Applied externally, this naturally fine clay eliminates toxins from the body, helps skin injuries heal and stimulates the skin's metabolism—and so does this mask, which will ensure that your skin looks clear and clean.

When to Use It

For puberty-related pimples and acne.

How to Use It

Apply the mask two or three times a week. Using your fingertips, apply the mask to your face, avoiding the sensitive areas around the eyes and lips. Let dry for about 15 minutes. Remove the mask using a washcloth and plenty of warm water, without rubbing too hard. Afterward, apply your favorite daytime face cream.

Shelf Life

The mask doesn't keep, so stir together a new batch each time and apply it right away.

You Will Need

+ Small bowl
+ Large washcloth

2 tbsp	bentonite clay	30 mL
Pinch	salt	Pinch
	Olive oil	
2 tbsp	chamomile tea	30 mL

How to Make It

1. In a small bowl, stir together bentonite clay, salt and a few drops of olive oil.
2. Stir in chamomile tea, a little at a time, until you have a smooth, thick paste.
3. Using your fingers, check the consistency. If the mixture is too thin, the mask will run off; if it is too thick, it will be hard to spread.

Tip

Some pharmacies carry ready-to-use masks that contain bentonite clay.

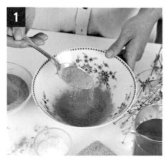

Combine bentonite clay, salt and olive oil.

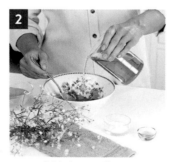

Add chamomile tea.

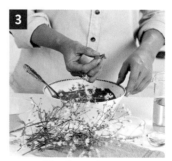

Check consistency.

Wound Cleanser

Marigold essential oil helps wounds heal by killing off bacteria, viruses and fungi. The beautiful, bright orange flowers (called pot marigolds or calendulas) often perform veritable healing miracles for all types of skin lesions, including nail bed infections, scars and abscesses. You have to try it to believe it!

When to Use It
For cleaning open wounds.

How to Use It
Wash the wound with the cleanser or place a compress moistened in the cleanser on the wound.

Shelf Life
The cleanser will keep for about 1 year in the fridge.

You Will Need
- Preserving jar (4 cups/1 L)
- Funnel
- Fine-mesh sieve
- Dark bottle (4 oz/125 mL)

0.35 oz	freshly picked marigold flowers	10 g
7 tbsp	70% ethyl rubbing alcohol	100 mL

How to Make It
1. Place marigold flowers in a preserving jar.
2. Pour ethyl alcohol over top. Seal tightly and place the jar in a warm spot. From time to time during the next 2 weeks, vigorously shake the jar.
3. Using a funnel and a fine mesh sieve, strain into a dark bottle, pressing flowers to remove liquid.

Tips
If you don't have fresh marigold flowers, make a simple cleanser by combining 20 drops calendula mother tincture (a homeopathic medicine available at some pharmacies) with 7 tbsp (100 mL) cooled boiled water, or 0.9% isotonic saline solution (also called sterile saline solution; look for it at pharmacies).

Look for 70% ethyl rubbing alcohol at drugstores. It is not the same as isopropyl rubbing alcohol.

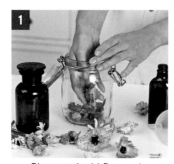

Place marigold flowers in preserving jar.

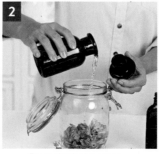

Pour alcohol over top.

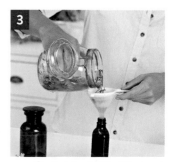

Strain into dark bottle.

Sage Candy

Sage is the classic medicinal herb used to fight sore throats and gum inflammation, and to treat the inside of the mouth or the throat. It fights the pathogens that cause illness and quickly soothes pain.

When to Use It

For sore throats.

How to Use It

If you have a sore throat, suck on a sage candy several times a day.

Shelf Life

The candy will keep for at least 1 year in an airtight container.

Tip

Ricola, the cough drop company, makes a sage candy with similar properties. Look for it at drugstores or online retailers.

You Will Need

- Sharp knife
- Cutting board
- Mortar and pestle (optional)
- Small saucepan
- Wooden spoon
- Baking sheet
- Parchment paper

| 10 | sprigs fresh sage (or 0.18 oz/5 g dried sage) | 10 |
| 3.5 oz | granulated sugar | 100 g |

How to Make It

1. Briefly rinse fresh sage under cold water, then lightly pat dry with paper towels. Pull leaves off stems. Using a sharp knife and a cutting board, chop sage leaves as finely as possible. (If you are using dried sage, don't rinse it, and grind it using a mortar and pestle.)

2. In a small saucepan, melt sugar over low heat, stirring constantly with a wooden spoon. Continue stirring until the sugar is light brown. Stir the sage into the sugar. Be careful: The water contained in the fresh sage leaves will make the mixture sizzle, bubble and spit. Making this candy is, therefore, not a job for children.

3. Take the saucepan off the heat. Line a baking sheet with parchment paper. Using a wooden spoon, drop candy-size portions of herb mixture onto the paper. Be careful: The sugar mixture is hotter than boiling water! If you don't like the shape of the candy, let the drops cool enough to handle, then, using your hands, roll them into balls.

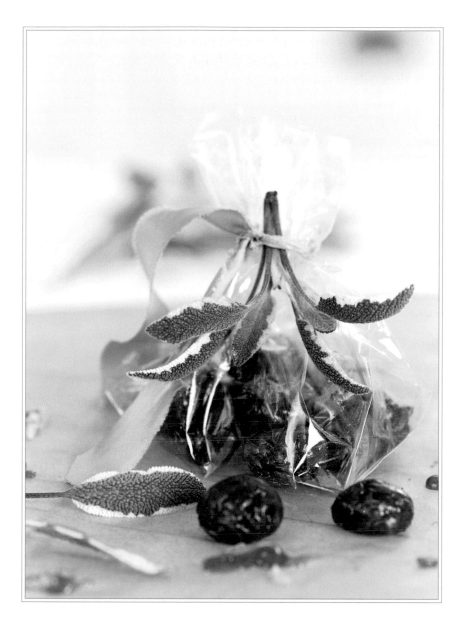

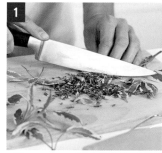

1

Chop sage as finely as possible.

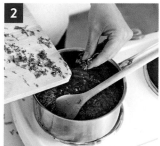

2

Stir sage into melted sugar.

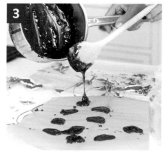

3

Drop spoonfuls of sage mixture onto parchment paper.

Pine Rubbing Lotion

Even by itself, spruce oil stimulates circulation, as in my Spruce Bath Salts (page 62). In this lotion, its benefits are combined with those of mountain pine, camphor and rosemary. A massage with this lotion brings quick relief and releases a wonderful pine-forest scent.

When to Use It

For sore or pulled muscles, bruises and painful joints.

How to Use It

Drizzle lotion into your cupped hand or directly onto the painful body part and rub or massage gently until it is absorbed. Pine Rubbing Lotion dehydrates the skin, so you shouldn't use it for longer than 1 week without a break.

Shelf Life

The lotion will keep for about 1 year in the fridge.

Tips

Some specialty stores, especially online ones that specialize in German products, carry ready-made versions of this remedy.

Rubbing alcohol comes in different types and concentrations at the pharmacy. Use the one indicated for best results.

You Will Need

- Funnel
- Dark bottle (about 4 oz/125 mL)

4 tsp	95% isopropyl rubbing alcohol (see tips, at left)	20 mL
50	drops rosemary essential oil	50
30	drops spruce essential oil	30
30	drops mountain pine essential oil	30
30	drops camphor essential oil	30
5½ tbsp	vodka	80 mL

How to Make It

1. Using a funnel, pour rubbing alcohol into a dark bottle.

2. Add rosemary, spruce, mountain pine and camphor essential oils. Pour in vodka.

3. Close the bottle and shake vigorously. The contents will turn milky, because the essential oils combine with the alcohol, creating an emulsion. As the lotion stands, the essential oils will return to the surface. To recombine them, vigorously shake the bottle before each use.

4. To use, pour the lotion into a cupped hand. Using your other hand, dip into lotion and spread over the affected area.

Caution

Never use Pine Rubbing Lotion before sunbathing, because it can make the skin more sensitive to UV rays. Also make sure that pine rubbing lotion only comes into contact with unbroken skin. Even on small scratches, it may cause a strong burning sensation.

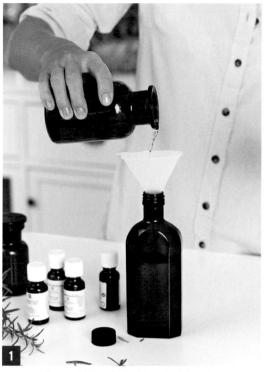

Pour rubbing alcohol into dark bottle.

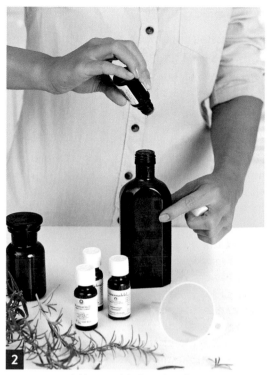

Add essential oils and vodka.

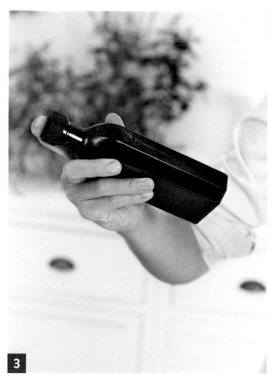

Shake well.

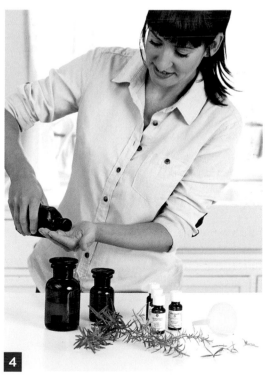

Pour lotion into cupped hand; use other hand to spread and apply oil.

Spruce Bath Salts

Only the young, tender shoots of the spruce are used in the natural pharmacy. An extract of these, used internally, helps expectorate mucus from the respiratory system; used externally, it stimulates circulation. Warm water further increases the effect of these bath salts. A pleasant side effect is that your bathroom will smell beautiful, like a walk in the woods.

When to Use It

For growing pains and muscular tension.

How to Use It

Add about 2 tbsp (30 mL) bath salts to a full bathtub of warm water. A bath in the evening before bed is particularly successful at treating children's growing pains, which usually occur in the evening or during the night.

Shelf Life

The bath salts will keep for 1 year in a dry place.

You Will Need

• Decorative resealable glass container (4 cups/1 L)

1½ lbs	sea salt	750 g
5 tsp	spruce essential oil	25 mL
1 tbsp	vodka	15 mL
	Green food coloring	

How to Make It

1. Pour sea salt into a decorative resealable glass container.

2. Add spruce essential oil and vodka.

3. Add food coloring as desired. Seal the container and, gripping tightly with both hands, shake vigorously back and forth, as if mixing a cocktail, to tint the salt.

Tips

You can add a little more spruce essential oil if you want an even more fragrant result.

Green food coloring gives the salts a beautiful color and is completely safe.

There are nice ready-made spruce bath salts available at some drugstores if you want to save time.

Caution

Spruce essential oil should not be used on children under the age of two years because it may lead to breathing difficulties. These bath salts are also not appropriate for children who suffer from asthma.

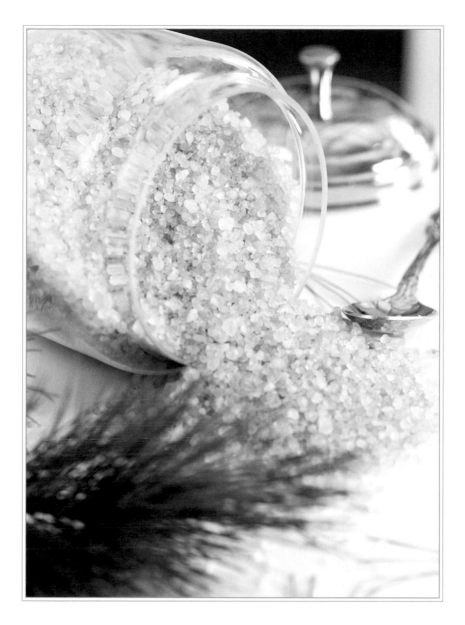

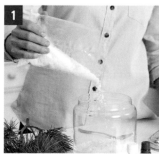

Pour sea salt into container.

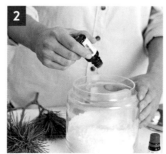

Add essential oil and vodka.

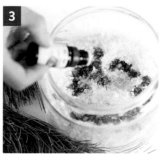

Color bath salts with green food coloring.

Coughs, Sneezes and Sore Throats

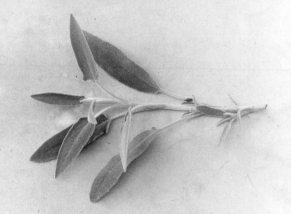

At some point during the winter, *it* will arrive. People will talk about nothing else—who's had it and who hasn't, and who's suffering from it right now. *It* is the flu. The accompanying fever, cough, sneezing, aches, pains, chills, shortness of breath and exhaustion make us collapse into bed, often for several days at a time. Fortunately, in many cases, when you feel unwell, you aren't dealing with the true influenza virus.

More often, it's a flu-like infection or a nasty cold that causes all that misery.

Yet what's the use of knowing this? You still feel terrible. Unfortunately, you might do whatever you can to protect yourself, but at some point cold viruses will still attack. And once they've made their home in your body, they have no objective other than to multiply.

Help from Nature

Nature has at its disposal a cornucopia of medicinal plants that can treat acute inflammation in the upper respiratory tract. Using these, you can fight coughs, sneezes, sore throats and their ugly companions in a gentle, effective way. "Nevertheless," you might say, "once I've caught a cold, I'll just treat it with something from the drugstore." I would advise against that. Why not simply go into your kitchen instead? There, in the crisper drawer of the fridge and in the pantry, you'll find cough syrup and nasal

spray. OK, not ready-to-use products, but the ingredients you need to make them.

And while you are calmly blending a gargling solution or brewing a cup of anti-flu tea, you're doing something else that is good for your health. Strength lies in finding peace. Stress weakens the body's immune system, offering germs a place where they can multiply. And at some point, while you are relaxing and enjoying a cup of your homemade anti-flu tea, that nasty cold will simply go away.

My Favorite Recipes for Treating Coughs and Sneezes

From the many herbs that fight colds, I have chosen the absolute blockbusters for their effectiveness. You can easily turn these into cough syrups and cold remedies.

Horseradish Cough Linctus (page 66)

Sure, horseradish is delicious with smoked salmon, baked potatoes and roast beef. But did you know that it is also a veritable bacteria and virus slayer? This cough linctus (thick syrup) is quite pungent and therefore not suitable for children, but it's effective in freeing the bronchi of mucus in adults.

Fennel Honey (page 68)

This is a gentle, soothing anti-cough remedy, made with wholesome organic honey, that is suitable for children and softies.

Sea Salt Nasal Spray (page 70)

Medicated nasal sprays from the drugstore act rapidly, but they also dry out the sinuses. Plus, your body quickly gets used to them, and you'll find it increasingly hard to breathe. This homemade sea salt nasal spray is much gentler. For extra help, rub Marjoram Ointment (page 37) under your nose when you use this spray.

Inhalation Mixture (page 71)

An inhalation is wonderfully effective at "blowing away the cobwebs" from your respiratory organs. This blend of eucalyptus, mountain pine and cajuput oils makes it especially effective.

Gargling Solution (page 72)

A tickly throat and difficulty swallowing are so bothersome—mostly because you simply can't scratch an itch deep inside your throat. This mix of sage tea, apple cider vinegar and tea tree oil will bring relief.

Anti-Flu Tea (page 74)

Meadowsweet contains the anti-inflammatory salicylic acid, which acts the same way in the body as the synthetic acetylsalicylic acid produced to make Aspirin. Need I say more? I warmly recommend you try this tea instead of popping a pill.

Expectorant Tea (page 75)

Maybe I should have given this tea a different name—mullein tea sounds a little nicer, doesn't it? On the other hand, now you know exactly what this tea does.

Irritable Cough Tea (page 76)

No matter how annoying it is, your cough won't be a problem; not even during a theater or orchestra performance, provided you drink this tea about an hour before.

Sinus Tea (page 77)

Besides meadowsweet, elder flower and lime, this tea also contains marjoram, myrtle, peppermint and echinacea. Being able to breathe freely through your nose is nothing to sneeze at!

Lemon Poultice (page 78)

You might not even want to think of lemons because they're far too sour. But they aren't if they're used externally in a poultice. Taken this way, even the most acidic lemon will banish the sore throat and painful swallowing that are causing you misery. It will make you happy again in no time.

Thyme Cream (page 80)

Thanks to its expectorant and antispasmodic actions, thyme should always feature in the Top 10 of cold-fighting herbs. Rub this cream on your chest, close your eyes, think of the ocean and breathe freely.

Horseradish Cough Linctus

The hot mustard oil in horseradish is its secret weapon. It kills off bacteria, fungi and viruses. Horseradish juice is an expectorant and strengthens the body's immune system, too. Because of these beneficial effects—and because of its rather rustic and hearty flavor—this spicy plant is also known as the "farmer's antibiotic."

When to Use It

For coughs, colds and bronchitis.

How to Use It

Take 1 tsp (5 mL) of the linctus three times a day.

Shelf Life

The linctus will keep for up to 6 days in the fridge.

You Will Need

- Vegetable peeler
- Grater
- Preserving jar (1 cup/250 mL)
- Funnel
- Fine-mesh sieve
- Dark bottle (8 oz/250 mL)

1	piece horseradish root (about 0.7 oz/20 g)	1
5 oz	organic liquid honey	150 g

How to Make It

1. Using a vegetable peeler and a grater, peel and coarsely grate horseradish root.

2. Place grated horseradish in a preserving jar and add honey. Seal the jar, place it in a warm spot and let it stand overnight.

3. The next day, using a funnel and a fine-mesh sieve, strain honey mixture into a dark bottle. Discard the solids in the sieve. Refrigerate the bottle until it is needed.

4. Take 1 tsp (5 mL) three times a day for coughs.

Caution

This cough syrup is not suitable for children because it is very pungent; for them, you'll find the perfect cough remedy in Fennel Honey (page 68). You should also avoid this remedy (and horseradish in general) if you are suffering from a stomach ulcer or an intestinal tumor.

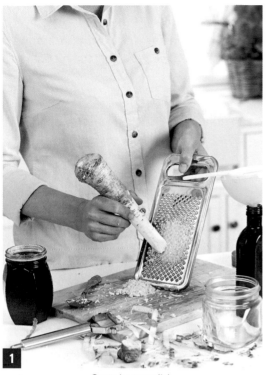

1 Grate horseradish.

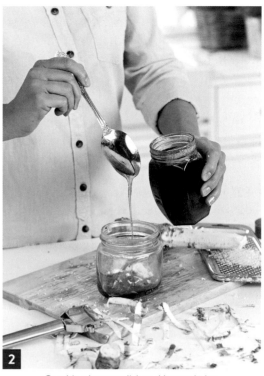

2 Combine horseradish and honey in jar.

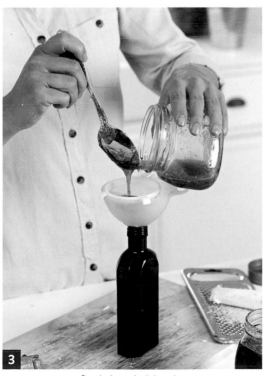

3 Strain into dark bottle.

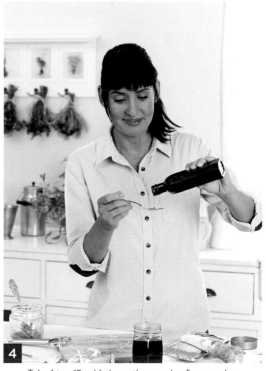

4 Take 1 tsp (5 mL) three times a day for coughs.

Fennel Honey

The active substances in fennel can loosen viscous mucus. Thanks to its antibacterial and antispasmodic properties, the plant also relieves digestive complaints and is therefore often used to treat babies and small children with upset tummies.

When to Use It

For a cold with a dry cough.

How to Use It

Take 1 tsp (5 mL) fennel honey three or four times a day.

Shelf Life

The fennel honey will keep for about 8 days in the fridge.

Tip

What sort of honey should you use? My secret is manuka honey, which you can find at high-end supermarkets and on the Internet. Its exceptional antibacterial properties have attracted the attention of scientists. However, studies of its medicinal applications have yet to be carried out.

You Will Need

- Mortar and pestle
- Saucepan
- Tea strainer
- Large teacup
- Preserving jar (2 cups/500 mL)

| 0.5 oz | fennel seeds | 15 g |
| 8 oz | organic liquid honey (see tip, at left) | 250 g |

How to Make It

1. Using a mortar and pestle, crush fennel seeds.

2. In a saucepan, combine crushed fennel seeds with 1 cup (250 mL) water. Bring to a boil. Strain the liquid through a tea strainer into a large teacup. Let fennel water cool a bit, then stir in honey—if the liquid is too hot, you'll lose the valuable enzymes in the honey.

3. Pour fennel honey into a preserving jar. Seal tightly.

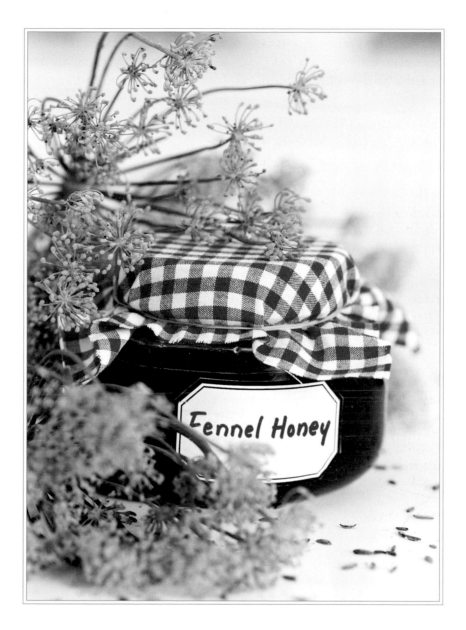

Fennel Honey

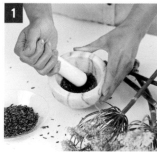

1

Crush fennel seeds.

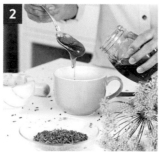

2

Dissolve honey in fennel water.

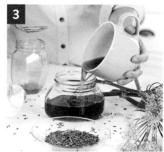

3

Pour mixture into preserving jar.

Sea Salt Nasal Spray

A solution made from natural sea salt (which isn't treated with bleaching or anticaking agents) moistens the sinuses and gently loosens the mucus associated with a head cold. This spray contains calendula mother tincture, a homeopathic remedy that is gently anti-inflammatory and antibacterial.

When to Use It

For a dry, stuffy nose.

How to Use It

Spray one or two squirts of the spray into each nostril as needed.

Shelf Life

The spray will keep for about 1 week.

You Will Need

- Large glass measuring cup
- Long spoon
- Small funnel
- Nasal spray bottle (1 oz/30 mL)

0.15 oz	natural sea salt	4.5 g
6	drops calendula mother tincture	6

How to Make It

1. In a large glass measuring cup, dissolve sea salt in 2 cups (500 mL) boiling water. (You will not need as much spray as this, but it makes it easier to weigh and achieve the proper ratio of ingredients.) Using a long spoon, stir until all of the salt crystals are dissolved.

2. Using a small funnel, pour sea salt solution into a nasal spray bottle.

3. Add calendula mother tincture, one drop at a time. Seal bottle and shake to combine.

Tips

This spray is also suitable for babies. Use an eyedropper bottle to administer it to infants, using one or two drops per nostril.

There are natural sea salt sprays available at pharmacies. Look for brands with no unnecessary additives.

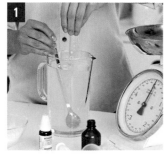

Dissolve sea salt in boiling water.

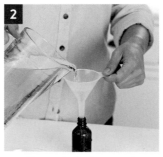

Pour solution into nasal spray bottle.

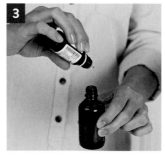

Add calendula mother tincture, one drop at a time.

Inhalation Mixture

You've probably heard that eucalyptus and mountain pine can help unblock the respiratory tract during a cold. But have you ever heard of cajuput oil? It is similar to eucalyptus, not only in scent but also because it contains exactly the same active substance: eucalyptol (cineole). The power of two is better than one!

When to Use It

For all cold-related symptoms: coughing, sneezing and a stuffy nose.

How to Use It

For inhalation, use six to eight drops for adults, or two to three drops for children over the age of 4 years. Inhale one to three times a day, for 5 to 10 minutes each time.

Shelf Life

The oils will keep for at least 1 year.

Tip

The mixture is also great to use in a cold-fighting bath. Combine six to eight drops with 2 tbsp (30 mL) cream and pour into warm bathwater.

You Will Need

- Dark bottle with eyedropper lid (½ oz/15 mL)
- Large bowl and towel (or inhaler)

½ tsp	eucalyptus essential oil	2 mL
¾ tsp	mountain pine essential oil	3 mL
1 tsp	cajuput essential oil	5 mL

How to Make It

1. Add eucalyptus, mountain pine and cajuput essential oils to a dark bottle with an eyedropper lid. Seal tightly and shake vigorously.

2. To make an inhalation, pour 4 cups (1 L) boiling water into a large bowl.

3. Add the recommended number of drops of the oil mixture depending on the age of the user (see How to Use It, at left). Drape towel over head and inhale steam.

Caution

The mixture is not suitable for children under the age of 4 years.

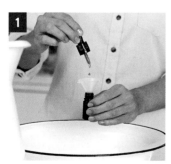

Drip essential oils into eyedropper bottle.

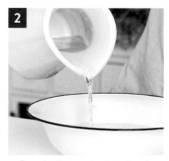

Pour boiling water into bowl.

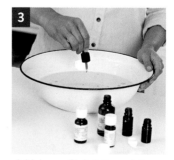

Add drops of inhalation mixture.

Gargling Solution

If your throat is sore or your voice husky, bacteria are usually to blame. A bacteria-killing gargling solution, such as one that contains sage, brings the quickest relief. It tastes quite medicinal, but you're not meant to drink it, after all.

When to Use It

For sore throat and hoarseness.

How to Use It

Gargle with this solution once every hour so that pain subsides quickly.

Shelf Life

The gargling solution will keep for 2 days in the fridge.

You Will Need

♦ Large pitcher, carafe or teapot

¾ cup + 2 tbsp	apple cider vinegar	200 mL
1¼ cups	cooled sage tea (brewed from fresh or dried sage), see tips, below	300 mL
10	drops tea tree essential oil	10

How to Make It

1. Pour apple cider vinegar and sage tea into a large glass pitcher.

2. Add tea tree essential oil.

3. Stir vigorously several times.

4. Gargle as needed, up to once per hour.

Tips

Why exactly is it that gargling soothes sore throats? It helps you achieve two things: First, the mouth and throat area are disinfected and bacteria are sent running; second, the sinuses calm down and swelling recedes, which, in turn, reduces pain. This solution is particularly effective if you tackle the bacteria in your throat simultaneously from the inside and the outside. I therefore warmly advise you to use the Lemon Poultice (page 78) at the same time.

A simple sage tea on its own makes a good gargling substitute for this recipe. For tea-brewing instructions, see page 21.

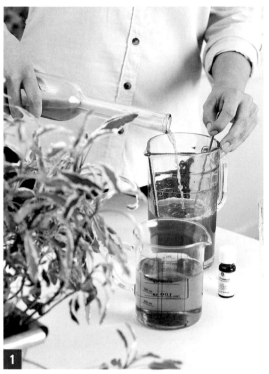

1 Pour apple cider vinegar and sage tea into pitcher.

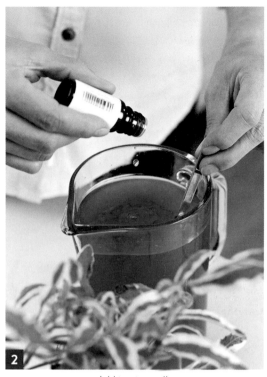

2 Add tea tree oil.

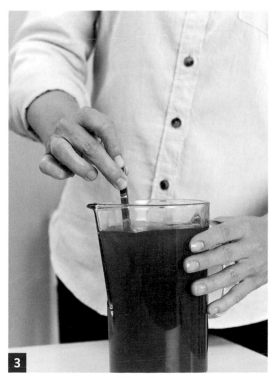

3 Stir well.

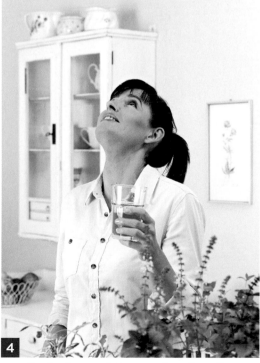

4 Gargle when needed, once an hour if you like.

Anti-Flu Tea

Meadowsweet contains salicylic acid and is therefore also known as "herbal Aspirin." It reduces fevers and soothes headaches and painful joints. Lime flowers and elder flowers support and complement this action. The best part: This tea has such a delicious aroma, you'll feel better just smelling it.

When to Use It

For colds with fever, and flu with joint pain.

How to Use It

Drink several cups of the tea over the course of a day.

Shelf Life

The tea mixture will keep for about 1 year in an airtight container.

You Will Need

- Tea caddy
- Tea strainer
- Teacup or teapot
- Thermos

1.8 oz	dried meadowsweet	50 g
1.8 oz	dried elder flowers	50 g
1.8 oz	dried lime flowers	50 g

How to Make It

1. Spoon meadowsweet, elder flowers and lime flowers into a tea caddy. Close the lid and shake vigorously to combine.

2. Place 1 tsp (5 mL) herb mixture in a tea strainer inside a teacup. Pour boiling water over top. (Alternatively, place 2 tbsp/30 mL herb mixture into a teapot and pour 4 cups/1 L boiling water over top.) Cover and let steep for 10 minutes. Strain into a Thermos.

3. Drink several cups over the course of the day.

Caution

Don't drink this tea if you are allergic to acetylsalicylic acid (the active ingredient in Aspirin).

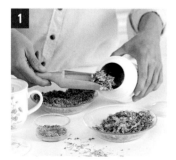
Combine herbs in tea caddy.

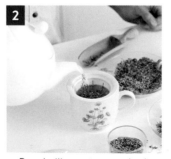
Pour boiling water over herb mixture in teacup.

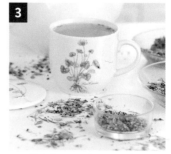
Drink several cups a day.

Expectorant Tea

Wild thyme, our kitchen herb's "wild brother," loosens mucus and ensures that it can be coughed up. It also kills off bacteria and viruses. Cowslip, mullein and aniseed also help thin mucus and make it easier to eliminate, plus they relax the respiratory tract.

When to Use It

For a stubborn cough with viscous mucus that cannot be coughed up (or only with difficulty).

How to Use It

Drink up to four cups of the tea over the course of a day.

Shelf Life

The tea mixture will keep for about 1 year.

You Will Need

- Mortar and pestle
- Tea caddy
- Tea strainer
- Teacup

0.7 oz	aniseed	20 g
1.4 oz	dried wild thyme	40 g
1 oz	dried cowslip	30 g
0.35 oz	dried mullein	10 g

How to Make It

1. Using a mortar and pestle, crush aniseed. Spoon crushed aniseed, wild thyme, cowslip and mullein into a tea caddy. Close the lid and shake vigorously to combine.

2. Place 1 tsp (5 mL) tea mixture in a tea strainer inside a teacup.

3. Pour boiling water over top. Cover and let steep for 10 minutes.

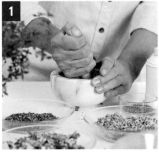

Crush aniseed using mortar and pestle.

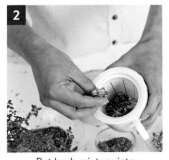

Put herb mixture into tea strainer.

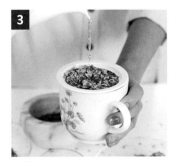

Pour boiling water over top.

Irritable Cough Tea

This herbal tea blend calms the irritated breathing apparatus without suppressing the cough reflex. The tea is not only exceptionally effective but also very mild, and is therefore suitable for infants. Most children like its sweetish flavor, and you can further improve on this with a little honey.

When to Use It

For a dry, irritable cough.

How to Use It

Adults can drink up to four cups of this tea per day. Children under 2 years of age should drink only about 2 tbsp (30 mL) daily (measure it in a baby bottle).

Shelf Life

The tea mixture will keep for at least 1 year in an airtight container.

You Will Need

* Mortar and pestle
* Tea caddy
* Tea strainer
* Teacup

0.35 oz	fennel seeds	10 g
0.9 oz	dried marshmallow root	25 g
0.7 oz	dried thyme	20 g
0.5 oz	dried ribwort plantain	15 g
0.35 oz	dried Iceland moss	10 g
0.35 oz	dried licorice root	10 g
0.35 oz	dried sweet violet	10 g

How to Make It

1. Using a mortar and pestle, crush fennel seeds.
2. Spoon crushed fennel seeds, marshmallow root, thyme, ribwort plantain, Iceland moss, licorice root and sweet violet into a tea caddy. Close the lid and shake vigorously to combine.
3. Place 1 tsp (5 mL) tea mixture in a tea strainer inside a teacup. Pour a generous ¾ cup (200 mL) boiling water over top. Cover and let steep for 10 minutes.

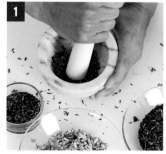

Crush fennel seeds.

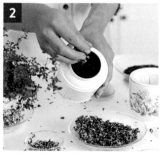

Combine herbs in tea caddy.

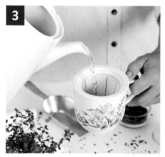

Pour boiling water over herbs in teacup.

Sinus Tea

The herb blend for this tea helps reduce the swelling of the mucous membranes and loosens mucus. It is also anti-inflammatory and strengthens the immune system. To intensify the benefits even more, you can use the infusion in an inhalation (turn to page 24 to find out what you'll need for that).

When to Use It

For paranasal or frontal sinusitis, as well as a stubbornly stuffy nose.

How to Use It

Drink up to four cups of the tea per day.

Shelf Life

The tea blend will keep for about 1 year in an airtight container.

You Will Need

- Tea caddy
- Tea strainer
- Teacup

0.7 oz	dried lime flowers	20 g
0.7 oz	dried marjoram	20 g
0.7 oz	dried myrtle	20 g
0.35 oz	dried meadowsweet	10 g
0.35 oz	dried elder flowers	10 g
0.35 oz	dried echinacea	10 g
0.35 oz	dried peppermint	10 g

How to Make It

1. Spoon lime flowers, marjoram, myrtle, meadowsweet, elder flowers, echinacea and peppermint into a tea caddy.

2. Place 1 tbsp (15 mL) tea mixture in a tea strainer inside a teacup.

3. Pour a generous ¾ cup (200 mL) boiling water over top. Cover and let steep for 10 to 15 minutes.

Caution

The meadowsweet in this tea mixture contains salicylic acid, so you should not use it if you are allergic to Aspirin.

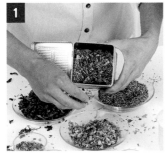
Combine herbs in tea caddy.

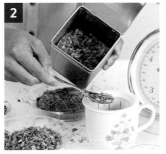
Spoon 1 tbsp (15 mL) into teacup.

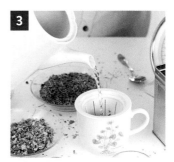
Pour boiling water over top.

Lemon Poultice

Not only do lemons contain plenty of vitamin C, but they're also rich in potassium, a mineral with antibacterial and anti-inflammatory powers. That makes this exactly the right remedy for a sore throat. If you also drink a cup of hot lemon water (see page 196), you'll feel much better quickly.

When to Use It

For a sore throat.

How to Use It

Let the poultice work for about 1 hour. During this time, you should rest. Afterward, remove the poultice, discarding the lemon slices. Then wrap a thin (silk) scarf around your neck and leave it in place for another 1 to 2 hours to protect you from drafts and the cold.

Shelf Life

The poultice can only be used once and a new one should be freshly prepared each time.

You Will Need

- Sharp knife
- Cutting board
- Tea towel
- Scarf

1	organic lemon	1

How to Make It

1. Using a sharp knife and a cutting board, cut lemon into generous ¼-inch (0.5 cm) thick slices.
2. Spread a tea towel across the work surface. Arrange lemon slices in a row lengthwise down the center of the towel.
3. Fold the long edges of the towel over the lemon slices to make a long, narrow package. Press down on the towel with your hand so that the lemon juice moistens the towel.
4. Wrap lemon poultice around your neck and hold in place with a scarf. Then, off to the couch with you!

Tips

If you feel a strong itch on your skin when you apply the poultice, immediately remove it and wash the affected area with plenty of clear, cold water.

Gargling with Gargling Solution (page 72) or a simple sage tea is a good complement to this poultice.

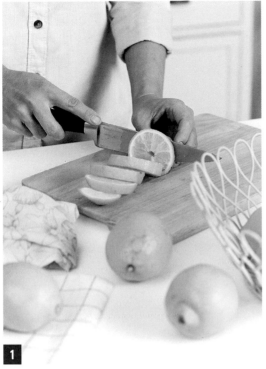

1 Cut lemon into slices.

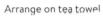

2 Arrange on tea towel

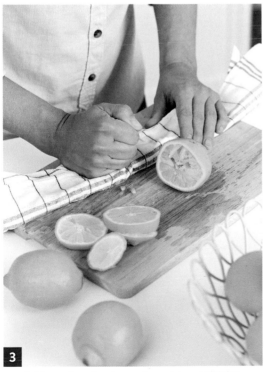

3 Fold over towel and press to moisten with juice.

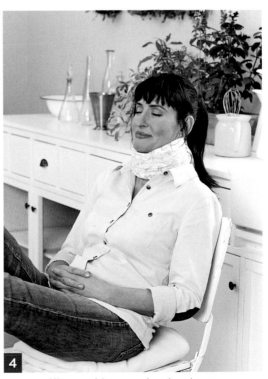

4 Wrap poultice around neck and rest.

Thyme Cream

Thyme is a disinfectant, antispasmodic and expectorant. This is why the herb has been used to fight asthma, bronchitis and whooping cough since antiquity. It also has a calming effect on the digestive system.

When to Use It

For acute or chronic bronchitis, spasmodic coughs and asthmatic breathing.

How to Use It

Gently rub thyme cream over the chest and back, both in the morning and before going to bed.

Shelf Life

The cream will keep for 6 months in the fridge.

You Will Need

- Sharp knife
- Cutting board
- Saucepan
- Spoon
- Thermometer
- Fine-mesh sieve
- Lidded jar

1	large bunch fresh thyme	1
8 oz	Melkfett (see tips, below)	250 g

How to Make It

1. Using a sharp knife and a cutting board, chop thyme as finely as possible.

2. In a saucepan, combine thyme and Melkfett. Heat mixture, stirring with a spoon, until it registers 104°F (40°C) on a thermometer. Once the temperature has been reached, take the saucepan off the heat and let cool. Each day for the next 7 days, reheat thyme mixture in a saucepan until it registers 104°F (40°C) on a thermometer, then let cool again.

3. On Day 8, after heating the mixture again, strain through a fine-mesh sieve into a lidded jar. Seal jar.

Tips

Strong essential oils, such as peppermint or eucalyptus, are frequently ingredients in cold-fighting creams and lotions used for chest rubs. If you are undergoing homeopathic treatment, these strong oils are taboo, because they can affect the action of the homeopathic medicines. This thyme cream doesn't contain them, however, and can be used in combination with homeopathic therapy without any problem.

Melkfett is a traditional German skin cream originally made to treat and protect cows' udders for milking. You can find it online and in some specialty stores.

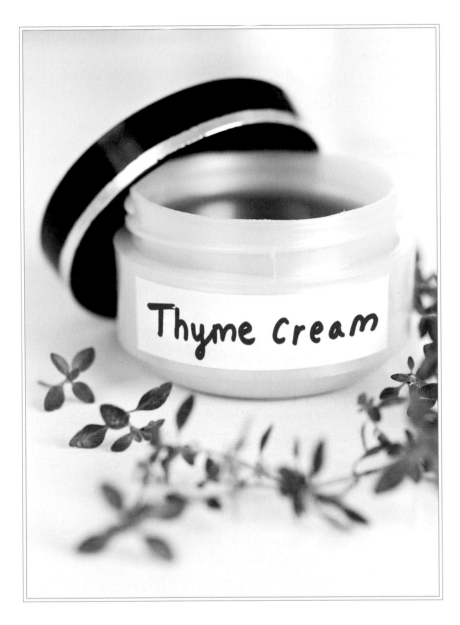

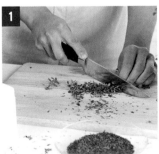

1. Very finely chop thyme.

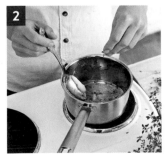

2. Heat thyme with Melkfett.

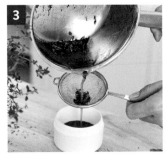

3. Strain through fine-mesh sieve into jar.

Stress, Go Away!

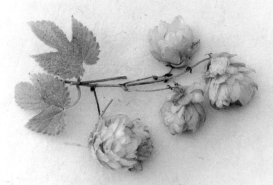

Here's a clear-cut case: If you're swimming in the ocean and suddenly everyone panics and runs out of the water—and everyone on the beach waves their arms around as if they've gone crazy—then this is, without doubt, a stressful situation. But, in truth, you don't need to borrow any scenes from *Jaws,* the classic horror movie, in order to explain the phenomenon of stress. Everyone has experienced stress. It is part of our lives, like our daily bread. When it comes right down to it, you could even say: He who has no stress is dead.

What Exactly Is Stress?

In fact, stress is simply a term for what happens in our bodies when we encounter extraordinary demands. When push comes to shove, we're able to unlock incredible powers—whether we have to escape from a shark whose fin is sticking out of the water or not.

Nor are the body's stress responses, as such, harmful to our health. Indeed, they are probably another reason why our species has managed to get this far at all. When our prehistoric ancestors encountered a sabre-tooth tiger or a hostile clan, their entire organisms would have concentrated on dealing with this problem. In order to do this, the brain would have activated a number of hormones, including both cortisol (hydrocortisone) and adrenaline. At the same time, the body would have attuned itself to maximum performance. The muscles would have been more efficiently supplied with blood, the blood sugar level would have risen, and hearing and sight would have become more acute.

Yet, whereas in the past stress was a relatively short-term condition—fight or flight (that is, movement) ensured that hormone levels would have dropped again quickly—today, we often run around like hamsters on a wheel. If stress is persistent or we do not get enough time between stresses to recover, body and mind will eventually sound the alarm bells and react to all that continuous pressure with so-called stress-related diseases.

Every body has its own preferred responses. One constantly sends its owner to the bathroom; meanwhile, another goes on an anti-digestion strike. Equally "popular" are tension headaches of all varieties, persistent fatigue, insomnia, heart and circulatory problems, and so on. It gets really serious when we're no longer talking about everyday stress but about high-caliber stress, such as the death of a close relative, divorce or an accident that causes profound anxiety. In these cases, consulting a physician becomes an absolute necessity.

Mostly, however, we're lucky enough to encounter only those types and forms of stress that are regular features of normal life. Nevertheless, we are expected to master these situations without any major theatrics. Therefore, I personally consider it legitimate to find some support. Some natural remedies will allow you to intercept those stress peaks, and others will help generate renewed energy.

My Favorite Recipes for Stress

During a period of stress, you don't just want to hope for better days to come—you want to make them happen within the shortest time possible. So I'd like to offer the recipes on the following pages to help ease your tense mind. The preparation is guaranteed stress-free! Oh yes—if, while browsing through this book, you miss the universally popular and tried-and-true Lemon Balm Spirit, go back and find the recipe in the What a Pain! chapter on page 94. It will protect you from sensory overload—and your stomach and intestines will also stop bothering you.

Heart and Nerve Tonic (page 84)

The ingredients for this mixture read like a *Who's Who* of tranquilizing herbs: valerian, hops, lemon balm and St. John's wort. No wonder then that this recipe has proved its worth even in the toughest, most stressful situations—times when I would normally not get a wink of sleep.

Healing Vinegar (page 85)

If stress is most likely to press on your stomach and you're one of those people who suffers from heartburn, I recommend this recipe. The bitter herbs in this curative vinegar mixture are a true medicine for the stomach. And because I use apple cider vinegar, it not only promotes healthy intestinal flora but also regulates your blood pressure. And, as we all know, blood pressure has a tendency to shoot sky-high during stressful times.

Rose Powder (page 86)

The lovely scent of the queen of flowers may not come to mind when you think of depressive moods—you may not think the two go together at all. Yet roses banish the blues. The positive effects of rose scent on the autonomic nervous system and a woman's hormonal balance has been scientifically proven. That means this smelling powder will have the same uplifting effect on your well-being as buying a whole closet full of brand-new designer stilettos. And if you compare the two, it's not even that expensive.

Anti-Stress Tea (page 88)

Lavender, sure. Hops, OK. But have you ever heard of holy basil? For centuries, the Hindu culture has regarded this herb as one of the most sacred plants, and as such it is an important component of Ayurvedic medicine. The list of its positive effects on health and well-being is indeed long. So it is hardly surprising that this exotic herb has been recognized as a true stress killer, even by modern science. You'll love it in this balancing drink.

Fenugreek Extract (page 89)

Thanks to the mucins it contains, fenugreek stimulates the appetite—and that's important for people who can hardly get a single bite down their throats due to stress. Your body will be even more weakened if you don't provide it with sufficient energy, and this recipe offers the help it needs.

Heart and Nerve Tonic

This recipe uses herbs that perfectly complement one another in their anxiety-reducing, relaxing and sleep-inducing effects. These plants are all tried-and-tested remedies, and their efficacy has been proven in a large number of scientific studies.

When to Use It

For anxiety, stress-related heart complaints and irritable colon.

How to Use It

Drink one liqueur glass per day, as needed.

Shelf Life

The tonic will keep for 6 months in the fridge.

Tip

Eau-de-vie is colorless fruit brandy (about 70% alcohol before distillation), usually made with any fruit other than grapes. Look for different flavors at your local liquor store.

You Will Need

- Large preserving jar (6 cups/1.5 L)
- Funnel
- Tea strainer
- Bottle (32 oz/1 L)

1.8 oz	dried passion flowers (or 3.5 oz/ 100 g fresh passion flowers)	50 g
1.2 oz	dried valerian root	35 g
1.2 oz	dried hop cones	35 g
0.9 oz	dried St. John's wort	25 g
0.9 oz	dried lemon balm leaves (or 1.8 oz/50 g fresh lemon balm leaves)	25 g
4 cups	fruit eau-de-vie (see tip, at left)	1 L

How to Make It

1. Spoon passion flowers, valerian, hops, St. John's wort and lemon balm into a large preserving jar.

2. Pour in fruit eau-de-vie. Seal the jar and place it in a very sunny spot. For the next 2 weeks, vigorously shake the jar once a day. To do so, grip it with both hands like a cocktail shaker.

3. On Day 15, using a funnel and a tea strainer, strain tonic into a bottle.

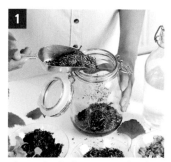
Spoon herbs into preserving jar.

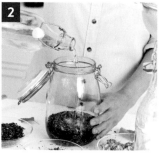
Pour in fruit eau-de-vie.

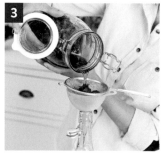
Strain into bottle after 14 days.

Healing Vinegar

I like to use vinegar as the base for herbal remedies. Apple cider vinegar is very healthy on its own, and if you add medicinal herbs that release their active substances into the liquid, it will become a veritable cure-all for all sorts of health complaints.

When to Use It

For heartburn, stomach pressure and a feeling of fullness. In addition, this healing vinegar helps detox, stimulates the immune system, balances acids and alkalis, has antibacterial powers and boosts metabolism.

How to Use It

To stimulate digestion, take 1 to 2 tsp (5 to 10 mL) healing vinegar in a glass of lukewarm water in the morning, on an empty stomach.

Shelf Life

The vinegar will keep in the fridge for 3 months.

You Will Need

- Funnel
- 2 dark bottles (each 32 oz/1 L)
- Tea strainer

1.8 oz	dried yellow gentian	50 g
1.8 oz	dried centaury	50 g
3 cups	naturally cloudy organic apple cider vinegar	700 mL

How to Make It

1. Using a funnel, spoon yellow gentian and centaury into a dark bottle.
2. Pour in apple cider vinegar. Seal bottle and place in a sunny spot for about 3 weeks.
3. Using a funnel and a tea strainer, strain vinegar into a clean dark bottle.

Caution

This healing vinegar is not suitable for pregnant women because it contains gentian.

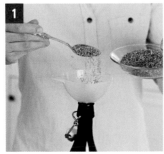
Spoon herbs into dark bottle.

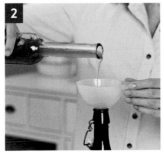
Pour in apple cider vinegar.

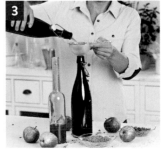
Strain into clean bottle after steeping.

Rose Powder

The rose is firmly established as a star in aromatherapy. Its perfume alleviates sadness, anxiety, fatigue and stress. And, as researchers at the University of Lübeck, Germany, have recently discovered, it also improves memory and makes it easier for people to learn.

When to Use It

For restlessness and to improve concentration; rose powder also has a calming and relaxing effect in stressful situations.

How to Use It

Carry a small jar of the powder around with you. Smell the contents as soon as you find yourself in a stressful situation or want to be able to concentrate better.

Shelf Life

Like all scents, the aroma of these herbs is volatile and will at some point evaporate. Over time, you'll need to replace the powder with a freshly ground mixture.

You Will Need

- Mortar and pestle
- Small lidded jar

0.5 oz	dried scented rose petals	15 g
0.18 oz	dried sage leaves	5 g

How to Make It

1. Using a mortar and pestle, grind rose petals with sage leaves as finely as possible.
2. Carefully transfer rose powder to a small lidded jar. Quickly cover with the lid so that the aroma cannot escape.
3. Open jar and inhale the aroma of rose powder to fight stress anytime.

Tip

Have some dried rose petals left over? Use them in a relaxing bath. The warm water releases the rose's essential oils so the petals can spread their beautiful perfume. And a rose bath for two by candlelight will win you romantic bonus points with your partner.

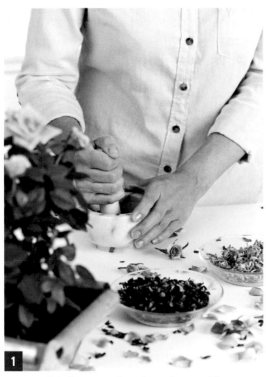

1. Grind rose petals and sage leaves with mortar and pestle.

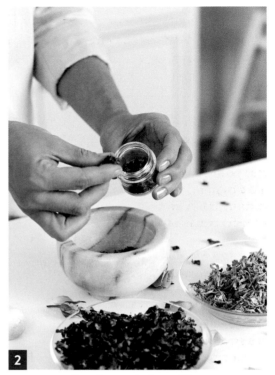

2. Transfer powder to small jar.

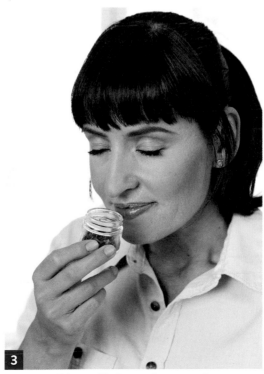

3. Take a sniff when you're stressed.

Anti-Stress Tea

Holy basil, known to Hindus as "the incomparable one," is an important medicinal plant in Ayurvedic medicine. It has also attracted the attention of scientists—studies have demonstrated that holy basil has soothing, painkilling powers that help people who suffer from stress, restlessness, digestive illnesses and cardiac complaints.

When to Use It

For balancing mood and alleviating stress.

How to Use It

In stressful times, drink several cups of the tea over the course of a day.

Shelf Life

The holy basil leaves will keep for 6 months in an airtight container.

Tip

Dried holy basil leaves can be a little harder to find than other tea leaves. Look for them in specialty tea stores.

You Will Need

- Teapot or teacup
- Funnel
- Tea strainer
- Thermos

| 1 tbsp | dried holy basil leaves (see tip, at left) | 15 mL |

How to Make It

1. Place holy basil leaves in a teapot (or use a smaller amount in a tea strainer inside a teacup, as shown in photo, at bottom).
2. Pour 4 cups (1 L) boiling water over top (or less for teacup). Cover and let steep for 10 minutes. Using a funnel and a tea strainer, strain tea into a Thermos and drink throughout the day (or drink as-is if using a teacup).

Caution

This tea is not suitable for pregnant women because the use of holy basil has not yet been scientifically researched in that situation.

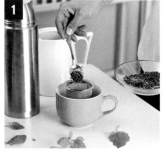

Place holy basil leaves in tea strainer.

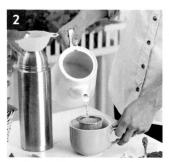

Pour boiling water over top.

Fenugreek Extract

For a long time, fenugreek was used mainly to treat burns. Today, it is also recommended for its invigorating effect; for example, to improve health after a long, enfeebling illness. It stimulates the appetite and supports the entire body during rehabilitation.

When to Use It

For lack of appetite.

How to Use It

To make use of the drink's invigorating effect, drink three cups of the cold extract daily over a period of 2 to 3 weeks. A word about taste: Medicine that works often tastes bitter, and fenugreek is a case in point.

Shelf Life

The finished extract will keep for 2 days in the fridge.

You Will Need

- Mortar and pestle
- 2 carafes or teapots
- Tea strainer

2 tbsp   fenugreek seeds   30 mL

How to Make It

1. Using a mortar and pestle, crush fenugreek seeds.
2. Spoon crushed fenugreek seeds into a carafe. Add 2 cups (500 mL) cold water. Let cold infusion steep for 2 to 3 hours.
3. Using a tea strainer, filter extract into a clean carafe.

Tip

Fenugreek stimulates milk production in lactating women. Drink a cup of the extract if you are producing too little milk and your baby is still hungry after breastfeeding.

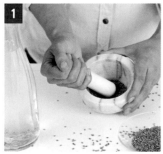

Crush fenugreek in mortar.

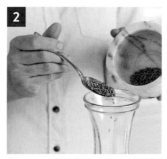

Spoon crushed seeds into carafe and fill with cold water.

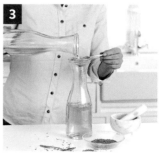

Strain into clean carafe.

What a Pain!

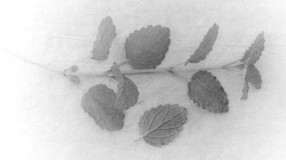

We all experience times when life seems to pass us by: Joy is a rare thing, nothing works and everything is simply a pain in the neck. Whether this is a brief spell of low spirits or a genuine crisis of the soul, it's hard to pull yourself out of the misery without any help. When psychological problems take on pathological dimensions, as in depression or burnout, lemon balm spirits or an ear massage won't completely fix the situation. But after taking my medicinal herb recipes, at least a ray of sunshine will pierce some of the smaller dark clouds.

For "Easy" Cases

When your mood is temporarily gloomy, you feel weak and despondent, and you can't rouse yourself to do anything, it's no reason to reach for pills—there are some amazing plants for precisely such cases. These remedies present you with a genuine alternative. They are generally well tolerated, have no side effects and don't make you dependent. Perhaps they don't act quite as rapidly as synthetic drugs, but if you regularly use these teas, tinctures and oils, your mood will soon climb back to its normal heights.

My Favorite Recipes Against Low Spirits

"There's nothing that cannot be cured by Lemon Balm Spirit," my grandma used to say. She knew, of course, that this statement was not an incontrovertible truth, but that wasn't the point. What Granny tried to say was that a positive attitude, confidence and a pinch of "don't-make-such-a-fuss-there's-a-solution-for-everything" are of the greatest importance for well-being and for getting back to full health. This sentence was therefore as much a part of the treatment as the Lemon Balm Spirit itself. When I smell it today, I immediately get a cozy, "everything's-going-to-be-all-right" feeling from my childhood.

St. John's Wort Tincture (page 92)

Many doctors recommend preparations containing St. John's wort to patients experiencing gloomy moods and those with depressive tendencies. And they are wise to do so—scientists have proven that this plant is just as effective as synthetic antidepressants. I recommend this tincture recipe as an alternative to teas and extracts in pill or capsule form.

Lemon Balm Spirit (page 94)

My grandmother's Lemon Balm Spirit really can do quite a lot. It helps fight migraines and tension headaches, stomach and intestinal complaints, menstrual problems, nervous heart conditions and colds. It's a balm for the stressed-out soul—literally.

Spring Tea (page 95)

Do you find it hard to drag yourself out of hibernation each year? Then make sure that, next spring, you try this tea. The blend of cowslip flowers, dandelion, stinging nettle, heartsease, speedwell and silver birch makes you feel like summer is just around the corner; plus it's extremely effective. By the way, the invigorating effects of this tea work other times of the year, too.

Lavender Oil (page 96)

This oil has a similar effect to that of my St. John's Wort Tincture (page 92). The reason is a substance called linalyl acetate, which is contained in the essential oil of lavender flowers. It has a calming effect on the central nervous system, making lavender oil a real mood enhancer. One noseful, and at least every second cloud will have a silver lining. It's a good mood to go.

Hangover Tea (page 98)

In Cologne, Germany, where I live, carnival (the so-called "fifth season") is firmly anchored in the annual calendar of festivities. I have my personal secret recipe for the day when all the frantic celebrations are over. (It helps me get used again to the fact that, in real life, I don't have red pigtails, nor is my name Pippi Longstocking). And that secret recipe is pu'erh tea. It's almost as fast to make as dissolving an old-fashioned fizzy tablet in a glass of water.

Hi There! Wake Up! Oil (page 99)

Aromatherapy makes use of many herb and fruit oils, because their scents have a positive effect on the mental state. This oil, with its lively explosion of aromas—cypress, rosemary, grapefruit and lemongrass—chases away gloom and listlessness. It'll revive the spirits of even the most fatigued souls.

Emerging from the Gloom

Activity in fresh air is certainly one of the very best measures you can take to raise low spirits. It stimulates the production of endorphins (happiness chemicals), and anti-stress hormones that occur naturally in the body, such as noradrenaline (norepinephrine). Don't worry—you don't have to morph into a top athlete to benefit from exercise. Just half an hour each day of brisk walking, gentle jogging or cycling is sufficient for you to reap these beneficial effects.

An added bonus of this "fresh air therapy" is the fact that you're exposed to plenty of natural light, which promotes the output of yet another happiness hormone, serotonin. At the same time, light inhibits the production of the sleep hormone melatonin. And this, by the way, is the reason why many people are especially listless and depressed in winter. During the winter months, we simply do not get enough natural light. "Light therapy" can help, and special daylight lamps are now available in just about every department store.

St. John's Wort Tincture

St. John's wort is the most frequently used phytotherapeutic treatment. One of the reasons for its popularity is the beneficial effect its active component, hyperforin, has on the messenger chemicals in the brain. This effect has also been verified by conventional medicine, too.

When to Use It

For depressive moods and anxiety.

How to Use It

For a very stressful situation that's not long-term, take 20 to 40 drops of the tincture in a little water as a one-off. Or try this tincture as a treatment over several months—in that case, add 20 to 40 drops to a glass of water and take once per day. In some cases, it may take several weeks for the tincture to fully develop its beneficial effects. Don't give up!

Shelf Life

The tincture will keep for about 1 year.

You Will Need

- Preserving jar (1 cup/250 mL)
- Small funnel
- Fine-mesh sieve
- Dark bottle with eyedropper lid (8 oz/250 mL)

2.1 oz	fresh St. John's wort flowers (or 1 oz/30 g dried St. John's wort flowers)	60 g
¾ cup + 2 tbsp	vodka	200 mL

How to Make It

1. Spoon St. John's wort flowers into a preserving jar.
2. Pour in vodka. Make sure the flowers are completely covered by the vodka so that they do not turn moldy. Seal the jar and place it in a warm, sunny spot for 4 to 6 weeks. From time to time, vigorously shake the jar.
3. Using a small funnel and a fine-mesh sieve, strain tincture into a dark bottle with an eyedropper lid.

Caution

St. John's wort increases the light sensitivity of skin, so don't take this tincture before sunbathing. This tincture may also interact with other medicines; consult with your doctor before using it if you are taking any medications regularly.

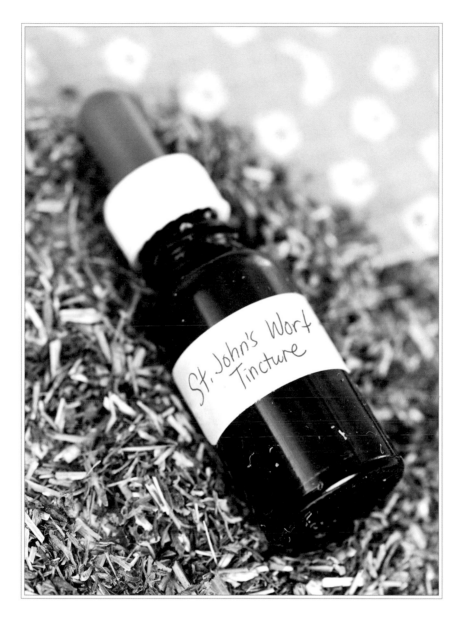

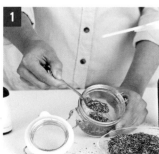

1 Spoon St. John's wort flowers into preserving jar.

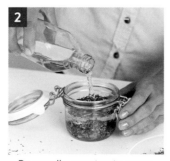

2 Pour vodka over top to cover.

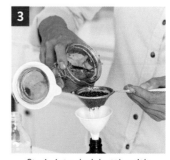

3 Strain into dark bottle with eyedropper lid.

Lemon Balm Spirit

Lemon balm, also known as Melissa, is one of the best known and most popular medicinal herbs around the world. This is due to the broad range of beneficial effects produced by its essential oils. In a nutshell, lemon balm has an all-around calming effect—on the stomach, digestive system, heart and nerves.

When to Use It

Internally, for nervous stomach and heart disorders, problems falling asleep, colds and as a tranquilizer; externally, for sore muscles, headache, gout and rheumatism.

How to Use It

Internally: Take 1 tsp (5 mL) Lemon Balm Spirit in warm tea or water (or with 1 tsp/5 mL sugar) one to three times a day. Externally: Apply undiluted to the skin.

Shelf Life

The spirit will keep for at least 1 year in the fridge.

You Will Need

- Large preserving jar (6 cups/1.5 L)
- Funnel
- Fine-mesh sieve
- Dark bottle (32 oz/1 L)

| 7 oz | fresh lemon balm leaves (or 0.35 oz/10 g dried lemon balm leaves) | 200 g |
| 4 cups | vodka | 1 L |

How to Make It

1. Place lemon balm leaves in a large preserving jar.

2. Pour vodka over top, ensuring that leaves are completely covered. Seal the jar and place it in a warm spot for 10 days. From time to time, shake the jar.

3. On Day 11, using a funnel and a fine-mesh sieve, strain liquid into a dark bottle.

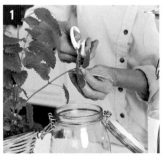

Add lemon balm leaves to preserving jar.

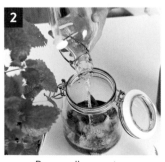

Pour vodka over top.

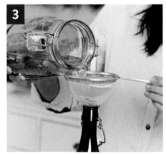

Strain into bottle after 10 days.

Spring Tea

As soon as the first rays of spring sunshine gently caress your face, you'll want to get rid of the winter blues—and that spare tire. All the plants in this tea, which are starting to grow this time of year, will help you do so. They're packed with vitamins, crank up the metabolism and help detoxify the body.

When to Use It

For springtime lethargy.

How to Use It

Drink a cup of the tea in the morning and in the evening every day during the spring.

Shelf Life

The tea blend will keep for at least 1 year in an airtight container.

Tip

This tea is an excellent supplement if you're fasting—its active substances detoxify and purify the body.

You Will Need

* Tea caddy
* Tea strainer
* Teacup

0.5 oz	dried dandelion leaves	15 g
0.5 oz	dried stinging nettle leaves	15 g
0.5 oz	dried heartsease flowers	15 g
0.5 oz	dried speedwell leaves	15 g
0.5 oz	dried cowslip flowers	15 g
0.5 oz	dried silver birch leaves	15 g

How to Make It

1. Spoon dandelion, nettle, heartsease, speedwell, cowslip and birch leaves into a tea caddy. Close the lid and shake vigorously to combine.

2. Place 1 tsp (5 mL) tea blend in a tea strainer inside a teacup.

3. Pour a generous ¾ cup (200 mL) boiling water over top. Cover and let steep for 10 minutes.

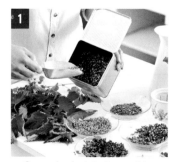
Spoon herbs into tea caddy.

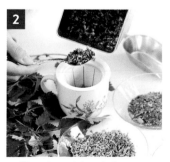
Place tea mixture in teacup.

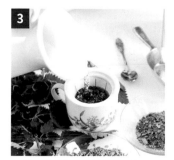
Pour boiling water over top.

Lavender Oil

Lavender—it conjures up lots of images. Some people will think of a sea of blooms in Provence, others will be reminded of their granny's lavender sachets in the linen cupboard. Everyone, though, will recall the same scent. It causes the brain to release more of the "happiness hormone" serotonin, encouraging relaxation. That "What a pain!" feeling will simply waft away.

When to Use It

For difficulty falling asleep, depressed moods and emotional tension.

How to Use It

If you want to forget the stress of everyday life and sleep more easily, I recommend a lavender bath. Stir 10 drops of this oil with 2 tbsp (30 mL) cream and pour the mixture into warm bathwater; this allows the lavender oil to blend into the water rather than float on top of it. A bonus is that the cream is tremendously good for your skin. For coughs or bronchitis, rub some lavender oil on your chest.

Shelf Life

The oil will keep for at least 1 year.

You Will Need

- Preserving jar (4 cups/1 L)
- Funnel
- Fine-mesh sieve
- Dark bottle (8 oz/250 mL)

2	handfuls fresh lavender flowers (or 3.5 oz/100 g dried lavender flowers)	2
¾ cup + 2 tbsp	almond or thistle oil	200 mL

How to Make It

1. Pull lavender blooms off stems and place in a preserving jar.
2. Pour in oil, ensuring blooms are completely covered. Seal the jar and place it in a warm, sunny spot for 6 to 8 weeks.
3. Using a funnel and a fine-mesh sieve, strain oil into a dark bottle, pressing blooms to extract oil.

Tips

If you need a mood lift, simply sniff the open bottle. You can also drizzle some lavender oil on a handkerchief and smell it from time to time when you're on the go.

A few drops of this oil on a fragrance lamp will fill the room with a calming, beguiling scent.

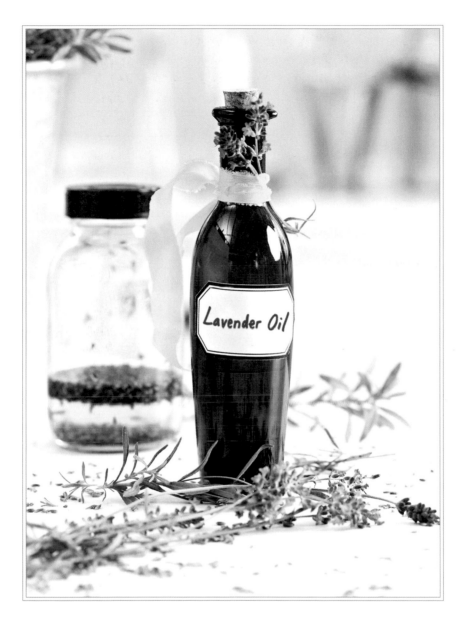

Lavender Oil

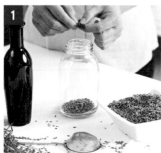

1

Pull off lavender blooms and place in jar.

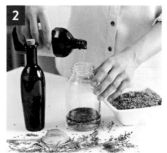

2

Cover blooms with oil.

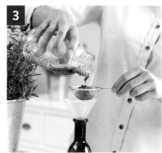

3

Strain into dark bottle.

Hangover Tea

A lot of positive things are said about pu'erh, a very old, traditional Chinese fermented tea. I particularly recommend this remedy for the typical side effects of a long night's partying. That's why it's my companion every year during carnival in Cologne.

When to Use It

For hangover symptoms, following the consumption of lots of alcohol.

How to Use It

Pu'erh tea contains caffeine, so you shouldn't drink more than three cups a day. You can reuse the tea leaves up to three times.

Shelf Life

In a tea caddy, the pu'erh tea will keep for at least 1 year.

You Will Need

- Tea ball infuser or tea strainer
- Teacup

| 1 tsp | organic pu'erh tea | 5 mL |

How to Make It

1. Spoon the pu'erh tea into a tea ball and suspend it in a teacup.
2. Pour a generous ¾ cup (200 mL) boiling water over top.
3. Depending on how strong you like your tea, let steep for 3 to 5 minutes.

Tip

Studies have indicated that many commercially available pu'erh teas contain excessive levels of pesticide residue. Make absolutely certain, therefore, that you use only organic tea.

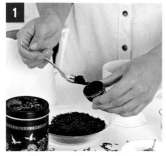
Spoon tea into tea ball.

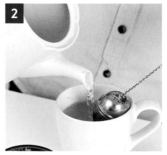
Pour boiling water over top.

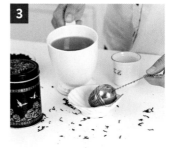
Steep tea for 3 to 5 minutes.

Hi There! Wake Up! Oil

This recipe gives you benefits two ways. The essential oils inhaled through the nose cause the brain to instantly switch into wide-awake mode. And an ear massage activates pressure points that improve concentration. This way, you'll have all your wits about you when it matters most.

When to Use It

For lack of concentration.

How to Use It

Inhale scent or use in fragrance lamp. For an ear massage, drop a little of the oil on your thumb, middle and index fingers. Knead the earlobe until it feels warm. Slowly knead along the outer rim of the ear to the top. One minute of massage is sufficient to make your ear feel warm and your spirit alert.

Shelf Life

The oil blend will keep for about 1 year.

You Will Need

- ◆ Small dark bottle with eyedropper lid (½ oz/15 mL)

¾ tsp	grapefruit essential oil	3 mL
½ tsp	cypress essential oil	2 mL
½ tsp	lemongrass essential oil	2 mL
¼ tsp	rosemary essential oil	1 mL

How to Make It

1. One after another, drip grapefruit, cypress, lemongrass and rosemary essential oils into a dark bottle with an eyedropper lid.
2. Seal the bottle and shake vigorously several times to blend oils.
3. Use as part of an ear massage for a quick concentration boost.

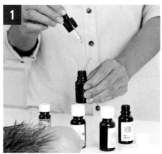
Combine essential oils.

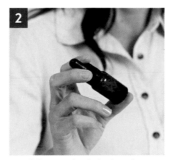
Vigorously shake bottle.

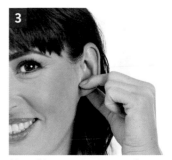
Use with an ear massage to boost concentration.

Women's Issues

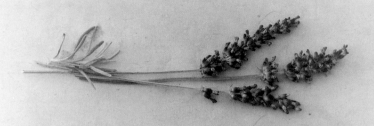

Herbal medicine and gynecology—for me, these two somehow just go together. And not just since it has been acknowledged that plant-based medicines are much easier to tolerate during menopause than the hormone therapies that have been liberally prescribed for years. After all, generations of women relied on their foremothers' knowledge of healing plants to treat the symptoms associated with this time of life.

Especially for Women

Polls have shown that women are much more likely to use natural medicines than men. This makes it worthwhile to look more closely at which medicinal plants are of special interest to women.

My Favorite Recipes for Women

Women and men are simply not made of the same material. And this is why I came up with a few very specifically "female" recipes. If you're looking for recipes for remedies to use during pregnancy, these are in the chapter starting on page 110.

Roll-On Lavender (page 102)

Women suffer from headaches and migraines more often than men do. Besides natural hormone variations, it's probably the female sex hormones that are to blame—they are believed to influence the way painful stimuli are processed. Also, changes in female hormonal balance can cause women to be more aware of stressful situations and to react to these with pain. Fortunately, nature has a multitude of plants that can help in such cases, so you won't always have to resort to pills immediately. One of these is lavender; this roll-on remedy made with it will protect you from all kinds of headaches.

Bearberry Leaf Tea (page 103)

Exposure to the cold can sometimes cause cystitis, and even the warmest pair of tights won't protect you when you're wearing your new miniskirt. You'll also be penalized with a bout of it in the summer if you run around for too long in a wet swimsuit on the beach or at the swimming pool. Some women even suffer from cystitis without having committed such "no-nos," and some have recurring episodes. In addition to keeping warm and dry, you should drink

There's the Rub

You don't need any brushes or rollers for an effective massage. Quite the contrary! (Many women perceive them as unpleasant anyway.) Simply make a fist, then allow your knuckles to glide over the skin in a circular motion while applying gentle pressure. Another good method is to hold a bit of skin with your thumb and index finger, pull it up, then release it again immediately, almost as if you were pinching yourself. Treat the entire affected area in this way, always in a circular motion.

plenty of bearberry leaf tea. It flushes out the urinary tract, and the active substances in this herb fight bacteria in the ureter, bladder and urethra.

Goji Berry Muffins (page 104)

Women usually want to look as slim and youthful as possible—and as long as they aren't obsessed with unrealistic models, this ambition is not, in itself, reprehensible. This muffin recipe will prove that foods that keep you looking good can also taste good. The muffins are made with a natural vitamin-packed miracle: the goji berry. Almost unimaginable amounts of vitamins, minerals and trace elements are present in this fruit: vitamins A, B_1, B_2 and C; iron; copper; nickel; chrome; magnesium; calcium; sodium; potassium; and amino acids. And that is just a short extract from a long list. So why do goji berries appear here instead of The Golden Age chapter on page 130? Well, I figure men will avoid this chapter like warm beer. And so the beauty secret remains where it should be—known to women alone.

Chasteberry Healing Vinegar (page 106)

A fundamental issue for women is the monthly period. This chasteberry healing vinegar has proven extremely beneficial for treating menstrual pain and premenstrual syndrome (PMS). It also helps more generally to readjust hormonal imbalances. But caution is advised: Taken over the long term, chasteberry can lead to lack of sexual appetite (an effect highly rated by

monks in the past, hence the berry's name). For this reason, it's best not to take this healing vinegar for more than three months at a time.

Skin-Toning Oil (page 107)

Cellulite, also known as orange skin by some, is, of course, not a purely female problem. But because of the gridlike structure of women's connective tissues, we just happen to be particularly prone to unsightly indentations on the bum and thighs. If cellulite puts you in a bad frame of mind, there's just one cure: massage, massage, massage. And this skin-toning oil—which contains the active substances in ivy, ground ivy and greater celandine—offers assistance.

Black Cohosh Tincture (page 108)

Many contradictory—and, unfortunately, worrisome—things have been said about hormone-replacement therapy as a treatment for menopause. You should therefore approach the subject with a critical eye and search, together with your gynecologist, for the solution that fits you best as an individual. The use of phytohormones (plant-based hormones) in black cohosh has proven to be an effective alternative to conventional hormone-replacement therapy. Its regulating effect on hormone balance is weaker—its phytohormones don't intervene as aggressively in natural processes. With this black cohosh tincture, you can see how well you adapt to phytohormones, generally without any worries.

Roll-On Lavender

The scent of lavender, as you already know from the previous chapter, can help the body release happiness hormones. Lavender is also very effective against headaches and mosquito bites. As a roll-on, it's a practical first aid kit that fits into any handbag.

When to Use It

For migraines and headaches, and to improve concentration.

How to Use It

As needed, rub the roll-on across the forehead and down the temples. If you find this too oily, roll over the neck and the insides of both wrists.

Shelf Life

The oil will keep for at least 1 year.

You Will Need

+ Small roll-on container (⅓ oz/10 mL)

2 tsp	lavender essential oil (or Lavender Oil; page 96)	10 mL

How to Make It

1. Pour lavender essential oil into a small roll-on container. Seal it up and it's ready to use.
2. Roll oil over temples as needed.
3. Or, if you prefer, roll over the insides of the wrists as needed.

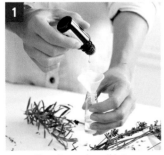

Pour lavender oil into roll-on container.

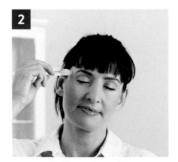

Roll over temples.

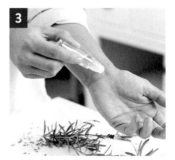

Or roll over insides of wrists.

Bearberry Leaf Tea

The naturally occurring components of bearberry have a strong antibacterial effect in the urinary tract. This cold water extraction method is recommended because the resulting tea won't irritate the stomach.

When to Use It

For cystitis.

How to Use It

If you suffer from uncomplicated cystitis, with the typical burning sensation during urination, drink one cup of bearberry leaf tea three times a day.

Shelf Life

The dried leaves or tea will keep for about 1 year.

Tip

If you can't find bulk dried bearberry leaves, some pharmacies and tea shops sell bearberry leaf tea, which is the same thing.

You Will Need

- 2 pitchers or teapots
- Fine-mesh sieve

2 tsp	chopped dried bearberry leaves or bearberry leaf tea (1.8 oz/50 g)	10 mL

How to Make It

1. Place bearberry leaves in a pitcher. Add 2 cups (500 mL) cold water. Let the extraction steep for 12 hours.

2. Using a fine-mesh sieve, strain the extraction into a clean pitcher. Now it's ready to drink.

3. Drink up to three cups a day. If you need urgent help, prepare the cold water extraction as described. At the same time, make a cup of bearberry leaf tea the "normal" way, with boiling water. Cover and let steep for 10 minutes. Drink the hot tea in small sips. Change to the cold water extraction when it's ready.

Caution

The active substances in bearberry are very strong and high doses may cause liver damage. Therefore, do not drink this tea for longer than 1 week at a time, and for no more than 5 weeks per year. This tea is not suitable for children under the age of 12 years, nor for pregnant or breastfeeding women.

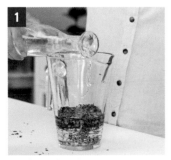

Steep bearberry leaves in cold water.

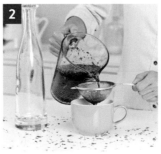

Strain extraction.

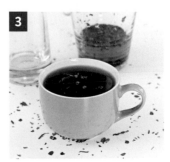

Drink up to three cups a day.

Goji Berry Muffins

Goji berries, also known as wolfberries, are considered a star among anti-aging plants. There's been no stopping their triumphal march since people found out that this superfood is the world's healthiest fruit. This recipe makes 16 muffins.

When to Use It

For high blood pressure and eye problems, and to support the immune system. The berries are supposed to slow down the aging process, as well.

How to Use It

Of course, these muffins taste best when they are fresh, but they're still good to eat a day later.

Shelf Life

Dried goji berries will keep for about 1 year in a cool, dry place.

You Will Need

- 2 bowls
- Whisk
- Wooden spoon
- Muffin pan
- Paper muffin liners
- Rack

7 oz	spelt flour	200 g
2.1 oz	rolled oats	60 g
1 tsp	baking powder	5 mL
½ tsp	baking soda	2 mL
2	organic eggs	2
6.3 oz	granulated sugar	180 g
5 oz	butter, softened	150 g
0.3 oz	vanilla sugar	8.5 g
10 oz	sour cream	300 g
7 oz	dried goji berries	200 g

How to Make It

1. Preheat the oven to 350°F (180°C). In a bowl, stir together spelt flour, oats, baking powder and baking soda.

2. In a second bowl, whisk eggs until foamy. Using a wooden spoon, continue stirring eggs. A little at a time, stir in granulated sugar, then butter and vanilla sugar. Stir in flour mixture and sour cream.

3. Gently fold in goji berries. Line cups in muffin pan with paper liners and spoon in batter. Bake in preheated oven for 20 to 25 minutes. Let muffins cool slightly in the pan. Transfer to a rack and let cool completely.

4. Enjoy muffins as a delicious, healthy treat.

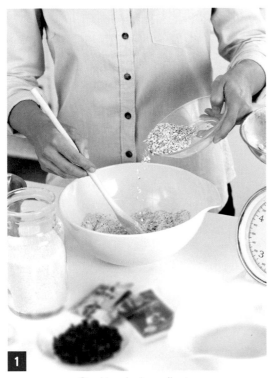

1

Combine dry ingredients.

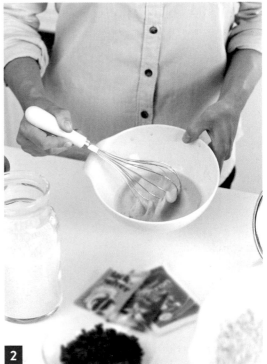

2

Whisk eggs until foamy.

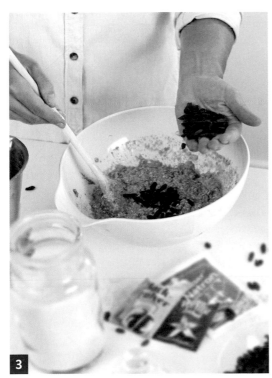

3

Fold in goji berries.

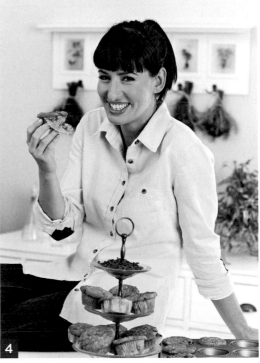

4

The taste of good health—delicious!

Chasteberry Healing Vinegar

Chasteberry helps with what used to be called "women's disorders," or cramps and PMS. In this recipe, it is assisted by lady's mantle and yarrow, which both have antispasmodic and calming powers.

When to Use It

For menstrual cramps and premenstrual syndrome (PMS).

How to Use It

Take 1 tsp (5 mL) healing vinegar per day. You can drink it either neat (careful—it's very acidic) or diluted in a little warm water and, if desired, sweetened with a little bit of honey.

Shelf Life

The vinegar will keep for 6 months in a cool, dark place.

You Will Need

- Preserving jar (1 cup/250 mL)
- Funnel
- Fine-mesh sieve
- Dark bottle (8 oz/250 mL)

1.8 oz	fresh chasteberries (or 0.9 oz/ 25 g dried chasteberries)	50 g
2 tbsp	dried yarrow	30 mL
2 tbsp	dried lady's mantle	30 mL
¾ cup + 2 tbsp	naturally cloudy organic apple cider vinegar	200 mL

How to Make It

1. Spoon chasteberries, yarrow and lady's mantle into a preserving jar. Pour vinegar over top, ensuring berries and herbs are completely covered.

2. Seal the jar, place it in a warm spot and let steep for 2 weeks. From time to time, vigorously shake the jar.

3. Using a funnel and a fine-mesh sieve, strain the vinegar into a dark bottle, pressing berries and herbs to remove liquid.

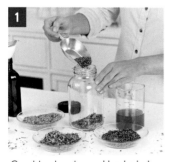
1 Combine berries and herbs in jar.

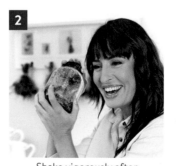
2 Shake vigorously after adding vinegar.

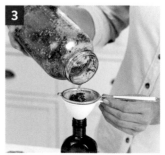
3 Strain into dark bottle.

Skin-Toning Oil

When applied externally, common ivy, ground ivy and greater celandine activate the skin's metabolism, promote waste elimination, and firm and smooth skin. Although an oil made with these herbs is not a miracle cure for excess weight, it will help firm the skin if you're on a diet.

When to Use It

For cellulite and to tone the appearance of skin.

How to Use It

Vigorously massage and knead oil over problem areas once or twice a day.

Shelf Life

The oil will keep for at least 1 year.

You Will Need

- Preserving jar (2 cups/500 mL)
- Saucepan
- Funnel
- Fine-mesh sieve or coffee filter
- Dark bottle (4 oz/125 mL)

1.4 oz	dried common ivy leaves	40 g
1.4 oz	dried ground ivy leaves	40 g
0.7 oz	dried greater celandine	20 g
7 tbsp	canola or other vegetable oil	100 mL
5	drops rosemary essential oil	5

How to Make It

1. Place the common ivy, ground ivy and celandine in a preserving jar. Place jar in a saucepan of boiling water.

2. Pour oil over herbs in jar. Seal jar and boil in pan for 15 minutes. Carefully lift jar with the hot herb and oil mixture out of the saucepan and place in a warm spot. Cover and let steep for 3 days, shaking from time to time.

3. Using a funnel and a fine-mesh sieve, strain oil into a dark bottle. Add rosemary essential oil. Seal bottle and shake to combine.

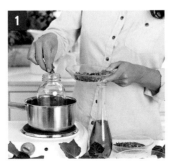

Put herbs into jar.

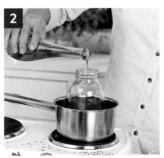

Pour oil over herbs and heat in water bath.

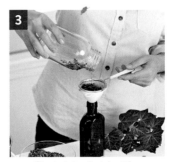

Strain into dark bottle.

Black Cohosh Tincture

Black cohosh has a similar effect on the female body as the hormone estrogen. It reduces the symptoms of common menopausal complaints.

When to Use It

For menopausal problems, such as hot flashes, sweating, disturbed sleep, nervousness and depression.

How to Use It

Over a period of 8 weeks, take 10 to 30 drops in a little water once or twice a day. The effect of black cohosh builds up slowly. In order to avoid undesirable side effects or habituation, take a 2-month break from the remedy after 8 weeks and change to a tea with a similar effect (for example, chasteberry tea from the pharmacy). Then you can go back to the black cohosh tincture.

Shelf Life

The tincture will keep for at least 6 months.

You Will Need

- Preserving jar (4 cups/1 L)
- Funnel
- Fine-mesh sieve
- Dark bottle (32 oz/1 L)

1 oz	dried black cohosh root	30 g
	Vodka	

How to Make It

1. Spoon black cohosh root into a preserving jar.
2. Pour in enough of the vodka to completely cover all of the root. Seal the jar and place it in a warm spot for 4 to 6 weeks. From time to time, vigorously shake the jar.
3. Using a funnel and a fine-mesh sieve, strain tincture into a dark bottle.
4. Add 10 to 30 drops to a glass of water and take once or twice a day.

Tip

Start this therapy as soon as possible after you first experience any problems, preferably in the first year of menopause. It's a good idea to talk to your gynecologist before you start taking this treatment. Have your hormone levels checked regularly when taking this tincture to ensure the proper balance is maintained.

Caution

If you suffer from breast cancer, check with your physician before trying this tincture. Black cohosh modifies hormone balance, which may not be beneficial in this case.

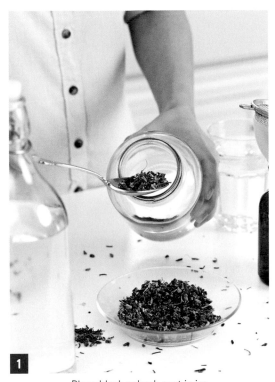

1

Place black cohosh root in jar.

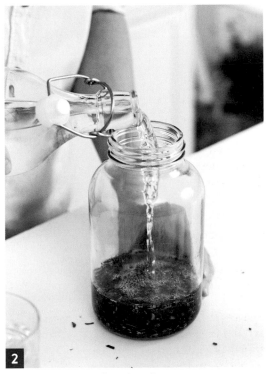

2

Pour in vodka.

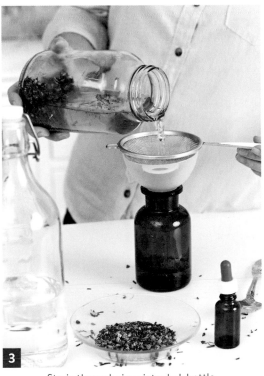

3

Strain through sieve into dark bottle.

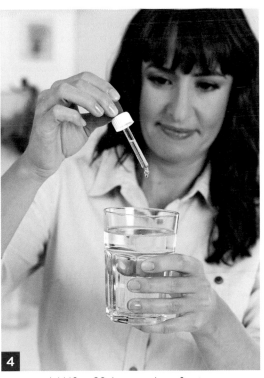

4

Add 10 to 30 drops to glass of water.

Baby on the Way

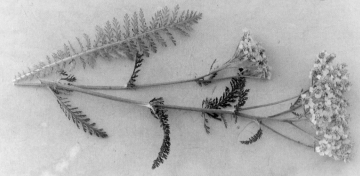

A baby's on the way—and along with it, unfortunately, comes nausea, vomiting, hemorrhoids, heartburn, stretch marks and so on. Luckily, it's a rare case indeed in which all these complaints appear at the same time. And hopefully you'll be happy to get through these things with a view to the wonderful time that awaits you after the birth of your child. If you take the long view, the small amount of discomfort really isn't worth discussing (too much). But when those symptoms are acute, there's nothing wrong with easing your suffering a bit.

Medicines During Pregnancy

Pharmaceutical drugs are largely taboo during pregnancy because of their potentially harmful effects on the unborn child. This is one of the reasons why, during these months, many women delve into the natural pharmacy when they normally wouldn't think of doing so. After all, there are many natural remedies that can effectively cure these unpleasant symptoms.

However, you still need to use caution with natural remedies. Some herbs can have unwanted effects during pregnancy, while other herbs need to be dosed differently during this time. If you are pregnant, make sure to take note of any special cautions on these pregnancy-related (and all other) recipes in this book.

My Favorite Recipes for Mothers-to-Be

Which problems, then, can you treat naturally with a clear conscience? You'll find them in this chapter. If you're also searching for a headache remedy without side effects, try Lavender Oil (page 96). Placing a cool cloth on the forehead and the back of the neck will also help, as will getting some fresh air.

Ginger Candy (page 112)
Ginger is a bit tricky: Too much of it may cause you to go into labor prematurely. On the other hand, though, it's the remedy of choice for fighting morning sickness. The answer is always the same: The dosage makes all the difference. At the right time, sucking on one of the ginger candies in this

chapter has never done anyone any harm; in fact, it has helped many a sick person. One caution: Even anti-nausea candies are still sweets and, therefore, should be enjoyed in moderation. That rules applies even more during pregnancy.

Potato Decoction (page 114)

You know that heartburn you get at the sight of fancy strollers? That could well be caused by their horrendous price tags, but the more likely culprit is the impaired locking mechanism between your esophagus and stomach. During pregnancy, especially the advanced stages, this ring-shaped muscle is weaker than normal. If the stomach pushes against it from below, it's easy for stomach acid to splash up into the esophagus. While there's not a lot you can do about affording the super deluxe version of your baby's first wheels, you can do quite a lot about those churning stomach acids. Just drink some potato decoction with caraway seeds for quick relief.

Anti–Stretch Mark Oil (page 116)

Personally, I think a child is a sufficient reminder of pregnancy. Why do you need stretch marks as well? (But who's asking me?) Luckily, you can—at least partly—control how accurately people can guess at your one-time incredible girth. I recommend you massage the areas at risk with this anti–stretch mark toning oil (try a brief pinching massage as well). After that, your skin will be so slippery that no stretch marks will stick to it.

Perineal Massage Oil (page 118)

If you start massaging the perineal tissue four to five weeks before your due date—preferably with this skin-conditioning oil—you'll be giving this sensitive area the best possible preparation for the exertions of delivery. Luckily, episiotomies are rare these days. This massaging may seem unusual at first, but it can help prevent tears in the perineum during delivery.

Breastfeeding Tea (page 119)

When your baby finally arrives, he or she will be hungry. Unfortunately, breastfeeding is not always as easy as expected. Many a new mom despairs because she can't produce sufficient amounts of breast milk. The psychological pressure of these demands can exacerbate the problem even further, because stress negatively affects lactation. However, this simple breastfeeding tea has proved successful in stimulating the flow of milk. Fenugreek, aniseed, fennel, lemon balm and lavender will help fill the "reservoir." The result is a baby in the land of milk (and honey), and a much-relieved mama.

Yarrow Balm (page 120)

Let's start at the bottom. I've heard of women who found labor pains less excruciating than the hemorrhoids that came later. (Just between you and me: Nature has arranged things so that later on, once it's all over, you can only vaguely recall those labor pains.) Hemorrhoids, small nodular piles around the anus, are not rare. Pregnancy hormones weaken connective tissue and dilate the blood vessels in the area. In addition, the expanding uterus presses on the veins in the rectum and causes blood to accumulate, so hemorrhoids grow larger. Constipation (hard stools) are common during pregnancy, and pushing during delivery can push those hemorrhoids outside. Yarrow is particularly soothing for this problem. It's the main ingredient in this balm—its active substances will ensure that your hemorrhoids disappear and that the irritated tissue no longer hurts.

Ginger Candy

Ginger strengthens the immune system, stimulates circulation, relieves cramps and thins the blood. This rhizome also relieves nausea and vomiting, which means that it is a popular remedy for motion sickness. It also helps many expectant mothers through the nausea associated with the first few weeks of pregnancy.

When to Use It

For morning sickness and motion sickness, but also for colds, sneezes and sore throats.

How to Use It

For morning sickness, starting at the first sign of nausea, suck on up to three candies per day. Don't take more than that because higher doses of ginger can induce labor. For motion sickness, suck on one candy about 30 minutes before starting your journey so that the ginger can take full effect.

Shelf Life

The candies will keep for about 4 months sealed in a tin lined with parchment paper.

Tip

These days, you can often find ginger candies made for exactly this purpose at drugstores.

You Will Need

- Sharp knife
- Fine small grater
- Small saucepan
- Wooden spoon
- Rack
- Parchment paper

| 1 | piece (1¼ to 1½ inches/3 to 4 cm long) fresh ginger (or more, to taste, for spicier candy) | 1 |
| 3.5 oz | granulated sugar | 100 g |

How to Make It

1. Using a sharp knife, peel ginger. Using a fine small grater, finely grate ginger to make 2 tsp (10 mL).

2. In a small saucepan, slowly melt sugar over low heat, stirring constantly with a wooden spoon. As soon as the sugar starts to turn light brown, stir in grated ginger. Take care because the mixture may splatter.

3. Take the saucepan off the heat. Line a rack with parchment paper. Drop candy-size portions of ginger mixture onto the paper. Be cautious, as the sugar mixture is very, very hot.

4. Let the drops cool slightly. Roll the drops between your hands to make a rounder shape. Take care, as the mixture will still be quite hot. Let the candies cool completely on the paper until hardened.

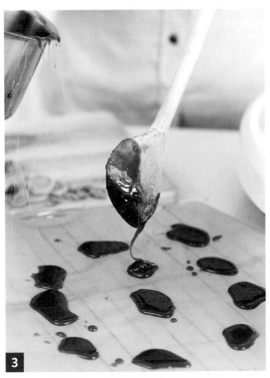

Finely grate fresh ginger.

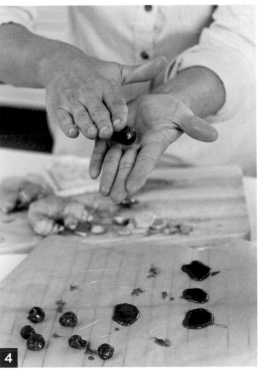

Carefully stir grated ginger into melted sugar.

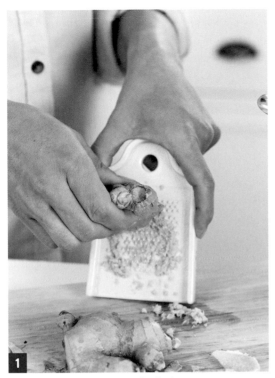

Drop mixture onto parchment paper.

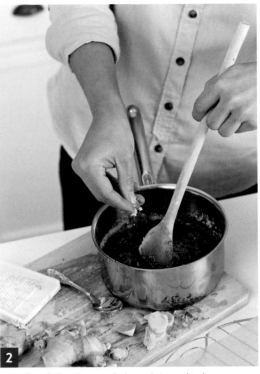

Roll candies into balls and let cool.

Potato Decoction

Many mothers-to-be swear by the antacid power of potatoes. During pregnancy, the steadily growing child presses on the stomach, making the locking muscle between the stomach and the esophagus "leaky." This allows stomach acid to flow back up into the esophagus, where it causes a burning sensation.

When to Use It

For heartburn and acid reflux symptoms.

How to Use It

Repeatedly drink a few sips of potato decoction over the course of the day.

Shelf Life

If you double this recipe, you can keep half in the fridge for the next day. The decoction will not keep for more than 24 hours, however, so use it up quickly.

You Will Need

- Vegetable brush
- Sharp knife
- Cutting board
- Saucepan
- Fine-mesh sieve
- Pitcher, carafe or teapot

1	small organic potato (any variety)	1
2 tsp	caraway seeds	10 mL
1 tsp	flaxseeds (not ground)	5 mL

How to Make It

1. Using a vegetable brush, scrub potato under cold running water. Using a sharp knife and a cutting board, chop (unpeeled) potato.

2. In a saucepan, combine 4 cups (1 L) cold (unsalted) water, potato, caraway seeds and flaxseeds. Cover and simmer over low heat for 20 minutes.

3. Using a fine-mesh sieve, strain the decoction into a pitcher.

4. Let cool to drinking temperature. Drink a few sips at a time throughout the day. And save the potato—you can eat it for lunch or supper!

Tip

Potatoes contain plenty of vitamin C, which is why they are also known as "lemons of the north." In addition, these tubers are rich in B vitamins, potassium, copper and folic acid, which is extremely important for pregnant women. Potatoes supply the body with carbohydrates and fiber, and contain virtually no protein or fat. In short, potatoes are the ideal health food to fill you up—as long as you don't eat them in the form of french fries, of course!

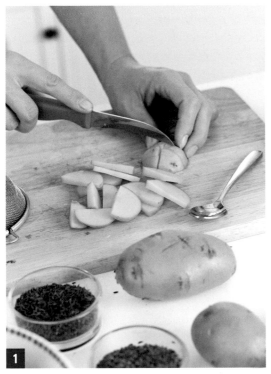

1

Chop potato.

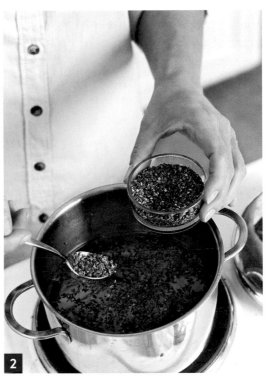

2

"Spice up" potatoes and water with caraway seeds and flaxseeds.

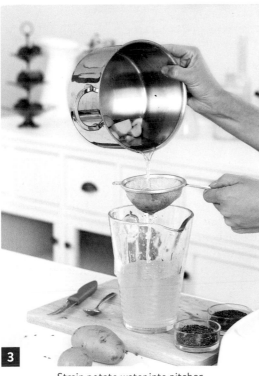

3

Strain potato water into pitcher.

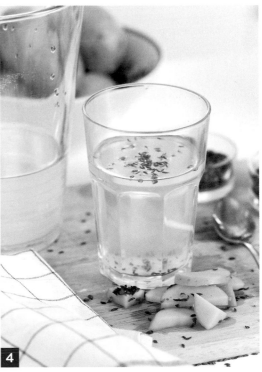

4

Let cool and drink a few sips at a time.

Anti–Stretch Mark Oil

During pregnancy, your skin has quite a lot of changes to cope with, especially around the abdomen. And so, it requires extra care. Rich avocado oil keeps the skin supple and promotes elasticity. An extra dash of vitamin E (the "skin vitamin") is a perfect complement to the oil, while gentle neroli and relaxing lavender essential oils give the mixture a heavenly scent.

When to Use It

For stretch marks.

How to Use It

Rub a little oil in your hands. Spread it over your belly wherever the skin feels tight. Massage it in.

Shelf Life

The oil will keep for at least 1 year.

You Will Need

- Funnel
- Dark bottle (4 oz/125 mL)
- Large sewing needle

7 tbsp	avocado oil	100 mL
10	drops lavender essential oil	10
6	drops neroli essential oil	6
2	vitamin E capsules (see tips, below)	2

How to Make It

1. Using a funnel, pour avocado oil into a dark bottle. (If the avocado oil already comes in a dark bottle, you can leave it and add the other ingredients to it.) Add lavender and neroli essential oils to bottle.

2. Using a large sewing needle, pierce vitamin E capsules.

3. Squeeze the contents of both capsules into the bottle. Seal the bottle and shake to combine.

Tips

A tendency toward weak connective tissue is genetic, but this oil allows you to improve the elasticity of your skin. It is particularly effective in combination with a daily pinching massage. Hold a small area of skin between thumb and index finger, briefly pull it up, then let go again. Work across all "tight" areas in the same way.

Look for gel capsules filled with vitamin E in the nutritional supplement section of the grocery store or pharmacy.

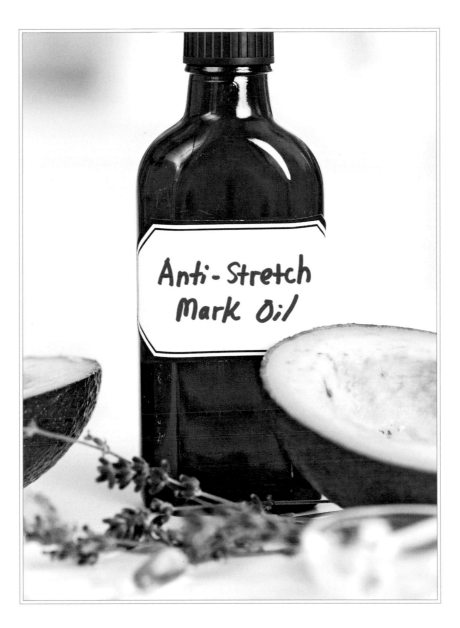

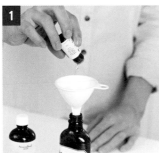

Add essential oils to avocado oil.

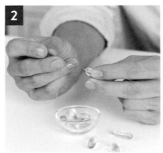

Puncture vitamin E capsules.

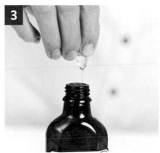

Squeeze contents of capsules into bottle.

Perineal Massage Oil

Many an expectant mother worries that her perineum (the area between the vagina and the anus) will not withstand the extreme challenge of birth and will tear. However, a good perineal massage oil helps you considerably improve the elasticity of that tissue during pregnancy, thus minimizing the risk of injury and the need for any surgical intervention.

When to Use It

For making the perineum more elastic in preparation for birth.

How to Use It

Put a little oil on your fingertips and gently massage the perineum for about 10 minutes. A daily massage is recommended starting at week 34 of your pregnancy.

Shelf Life

The oil will keep for at least 1 year.

You Will Need

- Small funnel
- Dark bottle (2 oz/60 mL)

2 tbsp	St. John's wort oil (store-bought or homemade; see page 52)	30 mL
4 tsp	wheat germ oil	20 mL
4	drops rose essential oil	4
2	drops clary sage essential oil (see tip, below)	2

How to Make It

1. Using a small funnel, pour St. John's wort oil and wheat germ oil into a dark bottle.
2. Add rose and clary sage essential oils.
3. Seal the bottle and shake vigorously to combine.

Tip

Clary sage *(Salvia sclarea)* is a member of the sage family, often grown to make essential oil. It has a nice fragrance and is often a component of massage oils.

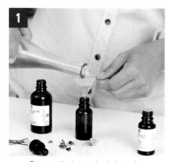
Pour oils into dark bottle.

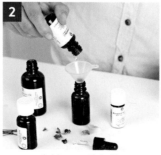
Add essential oils.

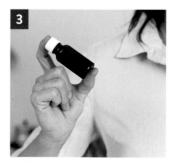
Shake vigorously to combine.

Breastfeeding Tea

You probably discovered fenugreek in the "Stress, Go Away!" chapter. Aniseed, fennel, lemon balm and lavender have also been mentioned in other places in this book. But have I told you that all of these herbs promote lactation in breastfeeding women?

When to Use It

For stimulating lactation.

How to Use It

Drink a maximum of two cups of this tea per day; if possible, one in the morning and one in the afternoon. The tea's action is intense and any more would make you overflow with milk. Only drink this tea if you feel that you really aren't producing enough milk. Otherwise, your body will get used to this "little helper."

Shelf Life

The tea blend will keep for at least 1 year in an airtight container.

You Will Need

- Tea caddy
- Tea strainer
- Teacup

0.7 oz	fenugreek seeds	20 g
0.7 oz	aniseeds	20 g
0.7 oz	fennel seeds	20 g
0.35 oz	dried lemon balm leaves	10 g
0.35 oz	dried lavender flowers	10 g

How to Make It

1. Place fenugreek, aniseeds, fennel seeds, lemon balm and lavender in a tea caddy. Close the lid and shake vigorously to combine.

2. Place 1 tsp (5 mL) tea blend in a tea strainer inside a teacup.

3. Pour boiling water over top. Cover and let steep for 10 minutes.

Tip

Pharmacies and health food stores often carry natural teas designed to encourage milk production. Try one if you don't have time to make this one from scratch.

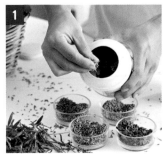
Combine seeds and herbs.

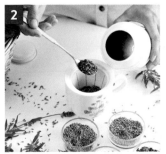
Spoon mixture into teacup.

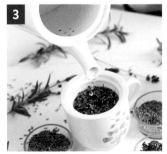
Pour boiling water over top.

Yarrow Balm

Taken internally, yarrow helps with "classic" women's complaints, such as vaginal discharge, menstruation problems and menopause symptoms. Taken externally, yarrow kills certain bacteria and has germicidal, anti-inflammatory and calming powers.

When to Use It

For hemorrhoids.

How to Use It

Apply a thin layer of the balm several times a day to hemorrhoids. It has a pleasantly cooling action and will quickly alleviate itching. To avoid transferring bacteria into the balm, make sure you thoroughly wash your hands before each use.

Shelf Life

The balm will keep for about 6 months in the fridge.

You Will Need

* Saucepan
* Wooden spoon
* Funnel
* Thin linen or cotton cloth (or clean cotton diaper)
* Lidded jar

3 oz	lard	90 g
0.5 oz	fresh yarrow flowers, chopped (or 0.28 oz/8 g dried yarrow flowers)	15 g
0.35 oz	dried red raspberry leaves	10 g

How to Make It

1. In a saucepan, melt lard, stirring with a wooden spoon.

2. Add yarrow flowers and raspberry leaves. Bring mixture to a boil, stirring. Cover the saucepan and take it off the heat. Let stand overnight. The next day, reheat the mixture.

3. Using a funnel lined with a thin cloth, strain mixture into a lidded jar. Let cool completely before sealing the jar.

Tip

If you don't have any of this balm on hand, you can also make a sitz bath with yarrow tea (add about 2 cups/500 mL tea to 20 cups/5 L water). It will help soothe hemorrhoids and menstrual cramps. If you soak your knee in it instead, it will help with arthritis in that joint.

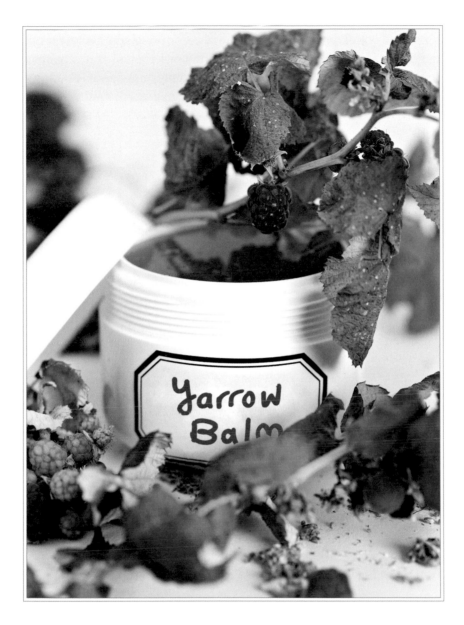

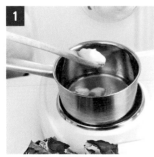

1. Melt lard.

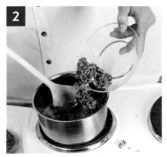

2. Add yarrow and red raspberry.

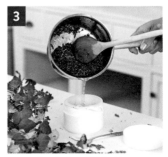

3. Strain into lidded jar.

Men's Issues

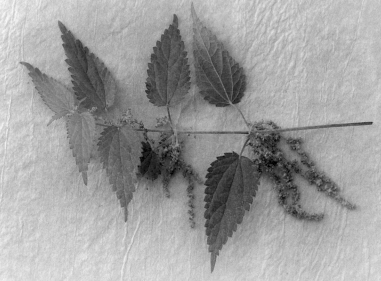

Men and health awareness—now that's a difficult topic. And I'm not at all surprised that men tend to use natural remedies considerably less often than women do.

Nevertheless, in this book, I didn't want to do without some select formulations for the opposite sex. Secretly, I live in hope that this may somehow change men's attitudes.

Natural Aphrodisiacs

Men are unlikely to discuss diseases or medicines in general, and are even less likely to discuss problems of virility, libido or the prostate (men like to think these problems only befall others). Despite that—or perhaps exactly because of that—most of my "men's recipes" deal with exactly these complaints. After all, herbal medicine

has quite a bit to contribute to this area. Natural aphrodisiacs fortify the sexual organs and improve sexual performance. For example, the scent alone of lovage, which is reminiscent of Maggi seasoning (a kitchen staple in many countries), is said to cause sexual arousal. And garlic and nettle seeds are believed to increase virility.

My Favorite Recipes for Men

Garlic may increase your sexual appetite, but the accompanying garlic breath can dampen your partner's eagerness. This is why I've created a few formulations without "aftertaste." Combined with a romantic bath for two or a tender massage, these remedies can genuinely do wonders.

Love Liqueur (page 124)

The aromas of cinnamon, lemon zest, thyme, coriander, mace and vanilla will transport you to a sensual world. Isn't it appropriate, then, that these spices will also crank up your interest in sex? This seductive recipe means nothing can stop you from

Male Menopause

Hormonal changes in the second half of life (better known as menopause) are not the sole domain of women; they also occur in men. The typical symptoms, such as hot flashes and disturbed sleep, do not become noticeable in men until later. Once they arrive, however, try taking a daily glass of water with a few drops of Black Cohosh Tincture (page 108).

enjoying 1,001 nights of sensual pleasure. And isn't it great that this home-brewed love liqueur has no side effects, unlike the well-known little blue potency pills? That'll make you twice as eager.

Virility Tea (page 126)

While we're on the subject, natural medicine can also do wonders when your nights of lovemaking are meant to not only bring you pleasure but also to produce offspring. The herbs in this tea increase virility and improve sperm quality—and thus the chances of your partner becoming pregnant.

Hair Tonic (page 127)

If your dad and grandpa were both bald, it's probably safe to say that their lack of hair was genetic. Unfortunately, there's no herb that can change that diagnosis. But for all other men, I recommend a regular scalp massage with this hair tonic. Stinging nettle, walnut and witch hazel all contain substances that supply nutrients to the roots of the hair, care for the scalp, and make the hair shiny and smooth. Plus, this tonic won't make your scalp itch, I promise!

Nettle Wine (page 128)

Reviving a tired man is not an easy task, but a pleasant glass of wine infused with stinging nettle can give him a new lease on life. After all, this herb, generally considered a bothersome weed, is exceptionally rich in vitamins A, B, C (twice as much as in lemons) and E; iron; calcium; potassium; magnesium; silicic acid; trace elements; chlorophyll; carotenoids; and flavonoids. Back in the days when fresh vegetables were scarce in the winter, people used to wait longingly for the fresh green leaves of the stinging nettle to emerge from the cold winter soil—it was one of the first herbs to do so. It allowed them to restock their bodies' vitamin and mineral deposits. If you don't want to get your nutrients from eating nettles the traditional way, simply drink a glass of this nettle wine. After four weeks, you'll feel ready to uproot trees, not just weeds.

Nettles in Soup

If you're one of the growing number of men who've discovered a passion for cooking, you can add the powers of stinging nettles to soup. In the spring, pick 2 handfuls of the tender shoots (wearing gloves, of course) and cook them in vegetable stock for about 10 minutes, adding 3 or 4 potatoes, finely chopped; 1 onion, finely chopped; and 1 clove garlic, chopped. Season with salt and pepper to taste, then purée the soup in a blender.

Love Liqueur

The components of this "miracle cure" act as natural aphrodisiacs—that is, they increase the blood supply to the male sex organs. The perfume of the spices in the liqueur alone will transport you to the realm of the senses, awakening your desire for love much better than a boring old blue pill.

When to Use It

For lack of sexual appetite and to increase sexual prowess.

How to Use It

Drink one liqueur glass; the mixture will start to work in about 30 minutes.

Shelf Life

The liqueur will keep for about 1 year in a cool, dark place.

You Will Need

- Large preserving jar (6 cups/1.5 L)
- Fine-mesh sieve
- Bowl
- Saucepan
- Wooden spoon
- Funnel
- Bottle (32 oz/1 L)

1	vanilla bean	1
0.7 oz	grated lemon zest	20 g
0.5 oz	dried thyme	15 g
0.35 oz	ground cinnamon	10 g
0.18 oz	ground coriander	5 g
0.18 oz	mace	5 g
4 cups	brandy	1 L
2 lbs	raw sugar	1 kg

How to Make It

1. Place vanilla bean, lemon zest, thyme, cinnamon, coriander and mace in a large preserving jar.

2. Pour in brandy. Seal the jar and place it in a very sunny spot for 2 weeks. From time to time, vigorously shake the jar. Using a fine-mesh sieve, strain the liquid into a bowl. Discard herbs and spices.

3. In a saucepan, combine sugar with 2 cups (500 mL) cold water. Cook over medium heat, stirring constantly with a wooden spoon, until sugar is dissolved. Reduce heat to low and continue simmering, stirring constantly, until the mixture has a syrup-like consistency. Add aromatized brandy and vigorously stir one more time to combine.

4. Using a funnel, pour liqueur into a bottle. Label bottle with recipe name.

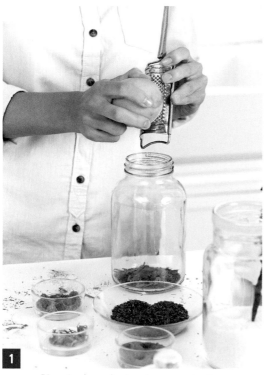

1 Place herbs and spices in preserving jar.

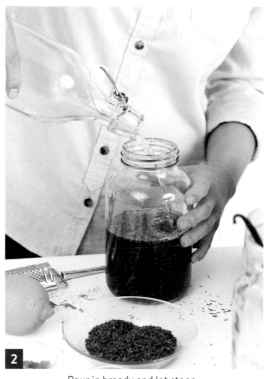

2 Pour in brandy and let steep.

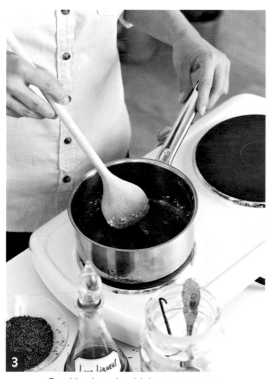

3 Combine brandy with hot sugar syrup.

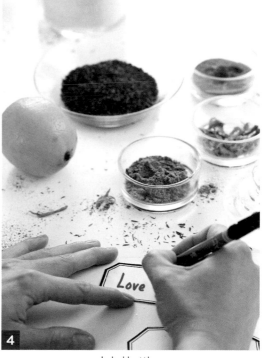

4 Label bottle.

Virility Tea

Speedwell, angelica and lovage roots crank up the metabolism and have a stimulating effect on the urogenital area. Parsnip also increases virility and fertility, and stinging nettle has a detoxifying and antacid effect, which is very important for the quality of sperm.

When to Use It

For improving sperm quality.

How to Use It

Drink one cup of the tea each morning and evening for 6 weeks.

Shelf Life

The tea blend will keep for at least 1 year. You'll just have to add fresh parsnip each time you make the tea.

You Will Need

- Vegetable peeler
- Sharp knife
- Cutting board
- Tea caddy
- Saucepan
- Fine-mesh sieve
- Thermos

1	piece (¾ to 1¼ inches/2 to 3 cm long) organic parsnip	1
0.7 oz	dried angelica root	20 g
0.7 oz	dried lovage root	20 g
0.7 oz	dried stinging nettle root	20 g
0.7 oz	dried speedwell	20 g

How to Make It

1. Using a vegetable peeler, peel parsnip. Using a sharp knife and a cutting board, finely chop parsnip. In a tea caddy, combine angelica, lovage, stinging nettle and speedwell.

2. Place 4 tsp (20 mL) herb mixture in a saucepan. Add 1⅔ cups (400 mL) water and bring to a boil. Add parsnip. Cover and simmer over low heat for 5 minutes.

3. Using a fine-mesh sieve, strain tea into a Thermos.

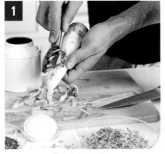
Peel parsnip.

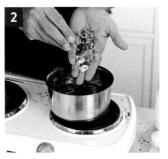
Bring water, parsnip and herbs to boil.

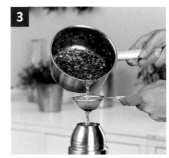
Strain into Thermos.

Hair Tonic

In this tonic, stinging nettle and walnut ensure that the scalp has good circulation, ensuring optimal blood supply to the roots of the hair. Witch hazel makes the hair shiny and smooth. If used regularly, this tonic prevents brittle and thinning hair the natural way.

When to Use It

For hair loss (not for hereditary or hormone-related baldness).

How to Use It

In the morning and the evening, massage a little hair tonic into your scalp. Just squirt a few drops straight from the bottle onto your scalp (or put a few drops into a cupped hand, spread it over the fingertips and apply to the scalp) and massage in.

Shelf Life

The hair tonic will keep for at least 6 months.

You Will Need

- Spray bottle (6 oz/175 mL)
- Small funnel

7 tbsp	witch hazel	100 mL
3½ tbsp	stinging nettle tincture	50 mL
2 tbsp	walnut tincture	30 mL

How to Make It

1. Unscrew the sprayer from a spray bottle. Place a small funnel in the bottle.
2. Pour witch hazel, stinging nettle tincture and walnut tincture into bottle.
3. Screw sprayer back on. Shake bottle vigorously to combine ingredients.

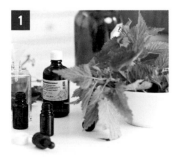
Prep spray bottle and ingredients.

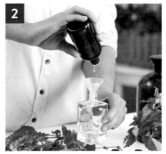
Put ingredients into spray bottle.

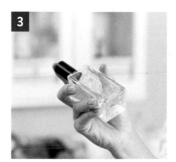
Shake vigorously to combine.

Nettle Wine

If you're tempted to write off stinging nettles as just a nasty weed that causes hives, you'll be doing them a very great disservice. For centuries, stinging nettles have been regarded as one of the most valuable medicinal plants. They are rich in vital substances, stimulate the metabolism, detoxify, promote blood formation and have anti-inflammatory powers.

When to Use It

For benign prostate enlargement; also for rheumatism, exhaustion and strengthening the elderly.

How to Use It

Drink one small glass of nettle wine in the morning and one in the evening for a period of 4 weeks.

Shelf Life

The wine will keep for 4 weeks in the fridge.

Tip

If you prefer an alcohol-free drink, prepare nettle tea instead. Pick a few fresh stinging nettle leaves (make sure you wear gloves!), put them in a teacup and pour boiling water over top. Cover and let steep for 7 to 10 minutes.

You Will Need

* Mortar and pestle
* Preserving jar (4 cups/1 L)
* Saucepan (optional)
* Funnel
* Fine-mesh sieve
* Dark bottle (32 oz/1 L)

1.8 oz	stinging nettle seeds	50 g
1	bottle (750 mL) good-quality white wine (preferably organic)	1
3.5 oz	organic liquid honey	100 g

How to Make It

1. Using a mortar and pestle, crush nettle seeds.

2. Place crushed seeds in a preserving jar. Pour wine over top. Seal the jar and let steep for 14 days at room temperature.

3. Add honey to wine. If it's not easy to stir in, warm the wine a little bit in a saucepan until the honey is completely dissolved. Using a funnel and a fine-mesh sieve, strain wine into a dark bottle. Discard nettle seeds. Seal bottle and refrigerate until needed.

4. Enjoy a glass of this aromatic drink once in the morning and once in the evening for 4 weeks.

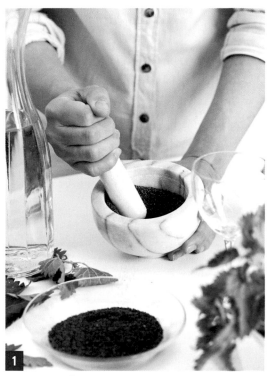

1 Crush nettle seeds in mortar.

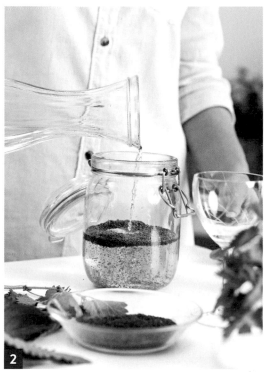

2 Place seeds in large preserving jar and top with wine.

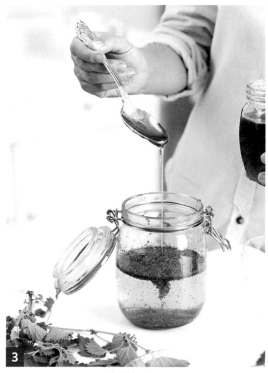

3 Add honey.

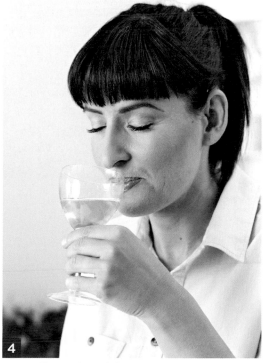

4 The result is a deliciously aromatic drink.

The Golden Age

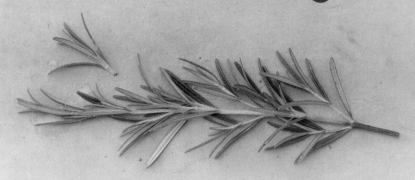

People are living longer lives, and, of course, everyone wants to enjoy this "bonus" time in the best possible health. Whenever the conversation revolves around this topic, I'm reminded of something that Hollywood legend Bette Davis once said: "Old age ain't no place for sissies." She was right. Like it or not, some limitations are part of the package that comes with the gift of growing older.

Staying Healthy to a Ripe Old Age

Since the body's self-healing powers, resilience and adaptability diminish over the years, it's important to preserve your quality of life for as long as possible. For this purpose, I recommend—you've probably guessed it by now—that you make use of the healing powers of nature.

Many older people can still remember how their own grandmothers treated minor (and even some major) health complaints with elder flower tea, leg compresses and onion bags. Perhaps this is why opinion polls confirm that seniors have an exceptionally positive attitude toward natural therapies. In addition, more and more physicians have recognized that medicinal plants and natural remedies can support conventional methods of treatment, mitigate side effects and sometimes even point to entirely new therapies. No wonder then that natural medicine is assuming an ever more important role in geriatric medicine.

My Favorite Recipes For Seniors

Herbal drinks, juices, wines…at first glance, the recipes in this chapter may imply that you can drink your way to a pleasant old age. But that's not really the case. Rather, these "youth drinks" are meant to contribute toward making you feel happy in your own skin for a long time to come. I would like you to take to heart my personal motto for getting older: "Stay relaxed in the face of what is to come, then take loving care of what you have."

Garlic Drink (page 132)
If you want to prevent high blood pressure, elevated cholesterol levels and arteriosclerosis (thereby reducing your risk

of heart attack or stroke), I recommend this magnificent remedy to you: garlic. Even if the pungent bulb is not your favorite, it cannot be praised highly enough for its health benefits. And don't worry—I'll also share a few simple tricks to help counter garlic breath along the way.

Rosemary Wine (page 134)

This recipe is a higher proof remedy; a merry wine, to be precise. Rosemary makes the blood flow hum along and steadies blood pressure, keeping it from falling into the basement. The herb makes everything circulate perfectly, so the brain can shift back to full power. Since this rosemary wine also tastes good, a little liqueur glass of it before bedtime can easily become a pleasant habit. However, it is a drug, so take a break after 2 months to avoid the much-talked-about habituation effect.

Rheumatism Tincture (page 136)

Millions of people around the world suffer from rheumatoid arthritis (RA), the most frequent form of chronic joint inflammation. Initially, those affected don't notice much change in their bodies. Perhaps they feel tired more often or their appetites decrease. Over time, however, the affected joints and the tendons that surround them become inflamed, making them hot, swollen or red. Worst of all, people who suffer from RA feel increasingly stiff in the morning. Rheumatoid arthritis cannot be cured, but with the help of anti-inflammatory medicines, physiotherapy, and heat and cold therapy, it can be kept in check. Diet is also of utmost importance. Those affected should, for example, eat as little meat and meat products as possible,

because the arachidonic acid they contain promotes inflammation. For acute pain, this tincture will help, with its inflammation-reducing and cooling properties. The simple act of paying attention to your body as you rub it on is also believed to be beneficial to your health.

Pomegranate Juice (page 137)

The pomegranate has been a symbol of beauty, fertility and power since time immemorial—it is therefore a symbol of youth. In the past few years, scientists have been able to prove that the active substances in pomegranates have amazingly positive effects on health. The most important and abundant are phenols. Among other things, they inhibit inflammation; protect the heart, blood vessels and brain; slow down cell aging; reduce high cholesterol; and even prevent cancer. I imagine that, in Hollywood, the home of ageless film stars, the cocktail of choice must be the pomegranate martini. Unfortunately, I don't have a recipe for that beverage, but I will reveal how to get the most juice out of this slightly obstinate fruit.

Herb of Immortality Tea (page 138)

Jiaogulan. Simply let the word melt on your tongue and enjoy the relaxation it brings. Then, when I tell you of all the things that this plant can do—strengthen the immune system, lower blood pressure and block free radicals—there will be no holding on to any stress. Known in English as herb of immortality, jiaogulan contains 50 more saponins (see page 186) than the other Asian cure-all, ginseng. A tea made from the herb is a veritable fountain of youth.

Garlic Drink

Garlic has a multitude of medicinally active substances, the most notable of which is allicin. This is responsible for its distinctive aroma; it is also the agent in garlic that kills bacteria and improves blood flow. There are even indications that allicin might clean up free radicals and prevent cancer.

When to Use It

For high blood pressure and high cholesterol, and to prevent arteriosclerosis.

How to Use It

Drink one shot glass full of the drink in the morning and in the evening.

Shelf Life

The drink will keep for about 1 week in the fridge.

Tip

If the pungent smell of garlic bothers you, simply chew on a leaf of fresh basil or a sprig of fresh parsley after taking the drink. This will quickly make your breath fresh again.

You Will Need

- Sharp knife
- Cutting board
- Blender
- Saucepan
- Wooden spoon
- Funnel
- Dark bottle (32 oz/1 L)

5	unwaxed organic lemons	5
30	cloves garlic	30

How to Make It

1. Using a sharp knife and a cutting board, trim off the ends of the lemons, then cut into thick slices. Peel garlic cloves.

2. In a blender, purée lemon slices with garlic.

3. In a saucepan, combine garlic mixture with 4 cups (1 L) cold water. Bring just to a boil, stirring with a wooden spoon. As soon as the mixture bubbles, take the saucepan off the heat.

4. Using a funnel, slowly pour the hot liquid into a dark bottle. Immediately seal the bottle.

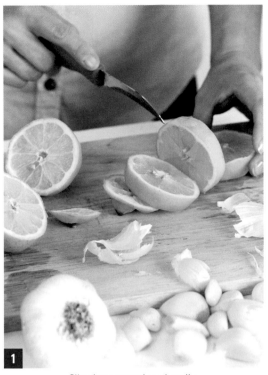

1 Slice lemons and peel garlic.

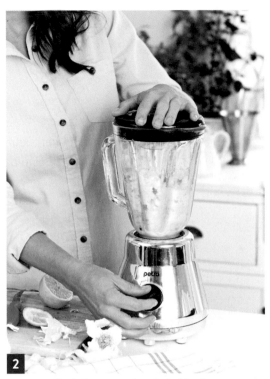

2 Purée lemons and garlic in blender.

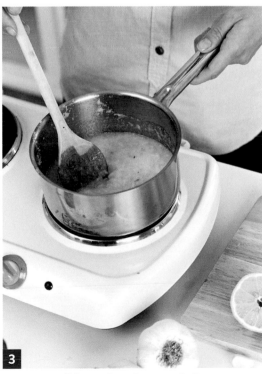

3 Bring purée and water to boil.

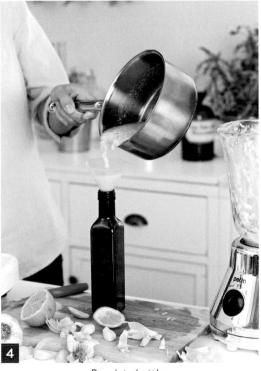

4 Pour into bottle.

Rosemary Wine

Rosemary calms the nerves, stimulates circulation and jolts the brain into action. This is why older people who suffer from low blood pressure can particularly benefit from this aromatic medicinal herb. Rosemary also brings quick relief for headaches and stomach cramps. Little wonder, then, that it was voted the medicinal plant of the year in 2011.

When to Use It

For improving memory, and to treat fatigue and headaches.

How to Use It

After your evening meal, drink one liqueur glass of rosemary wine. Take a 1-month break after 4 weeks so this evening drink doesn't become a habit.

Shelf Life

The wine will keep for 2 months in the fridge.

You Will Need

- Sharp knife
- Cutting board
- Funnel
- 2 dark bottles (each 32 oz/1 L)
- Fine-mesh sieve

5	sprigs fresh rosemary	5
1	piece (about ¾ inch/2 cm long) fresh ginger	1
1	bottle (750 mL) organic dry red wine	1
1	cinnamon stick	1

How to Make It

1. Pull rosemary leaves off stems. Using a sharp knife and a cutting board, chop rosemary leaves as finely as possible.

2. Using a sharp knife, peel and thinly slice ginger.

3. Using a funnel, pour wine into a dark bottle. Add rosemary, ginger and cinnamon stick. Seal the bottle, place it in a sunny spot and let steep for 2 weeks. Once a day, shake the bottle. Using a funnel and a fine-mesh sieve, strain the wine into a clean dark bottle. Seal and refrigerate until chilled.

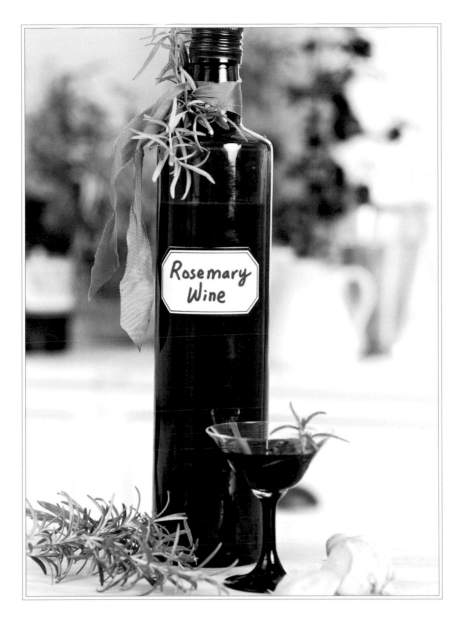

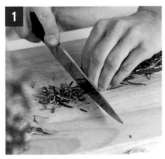

Finely chop rosemary.

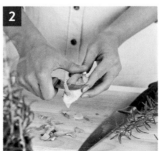

Peel and slice ginger.

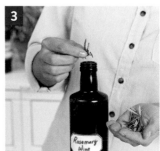

Combine ingredients in
dark bottle.

Rheumatism Tincture

*I've already conjured up the fabulously effective Pine Rubbing Lotion (page 60).
This tincture adds pine needles to that remedy, which makes it even more effective
for rheumatic pain. It is pleasantly cooling and penetrates right down to the painful
joint, where it alleviates inflammation.*

When to Use It

For aching joints caused
by rheumatism or gout.

How to Use It

For optimum results, rub
the tincture over painful
joints twice a day. It
quickly dehydrates skin,
though, so take a break
from this treatment as
soon as your skin begins
to feel tight.

Shelf Life

The tincture will keep for
at least 1 year.

You Will Need

* Preserving jar (4 cups/1 L)
* Funnel
* Fine-mesh sieve
* Dark bottle (8 oz/250 mL)

2	batches Pine Rubbing Lotion (page 60)	2
1.4 oz	dried pine needles (or large handful fresh young pine shoots)	40 g

How to Make It

1. Pour Pine Rubbing Lotion into a preserving jar.
2. Add pine needles. Seal the jar and shake vigorously to combine. Place the jar in a warm spot and let steep for 2 weeks.
3. Using a funnel and a fine-mesh sieve, strain tincture into a dark bottle.

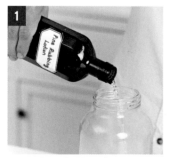

Pour Pine Rubbing Lotion into
preserving jar.

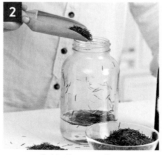

Add pine needles.

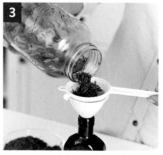

Strain into dark bottle.

Pomegranate Juice

Pomegranates contain three to four times as many antioxidants as red wine or green tea. They are therefore extremely effective at fighting arteriosclerosis and cancer. The best thing about this "apple of Aphrodite" is that its juice is absolutely delicious.

When to Use It

For cardiovascular diseases and joint complaints; and to prevent cancer.

How to Use It

Drink the juice whenever you want to do yourself some good—daily, if you like.

Shelf Life

The whole fruit will keep for several months in the fridge. Once the seeds have been removed, eat them right away.

You Will Need

- Cutting board
- Sharp knife
- Straw
- Small bowl and teaspoon (optional)

| 1 | pomegranate | 1 |

How to Make It

1. Press and roll pomegranate back and forth on a cutting board. You will hear a cracking sound when the seed coverings burst.

2. Using a sharp knife, make a hole in the top of the pomegranate.

3. Stick a straw into the hole and drink all the juice. If you'd also like to snack on the bittersweet seeds, cut the pomegranate open afterward, through the blossom end. Put the halves in a small bowl of water and, underwater, scrape out the seeds using a teaspoon. This will protect you from splashes of the tannin-rich juice, which makes tenacious stains on fabric. Simply fish the seeds out of the water when you're done.

Tip

These days, it seems like every store carries pomegranate juice, and it is a convenient, healthy drink to enjoy when you're on the go. Just choose a brand made with 100% juice (no added sugar); you'll often find bottles at health food or organic stores.

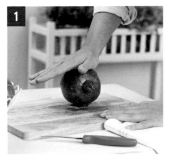
Roll pomegranate on cutting board several times.

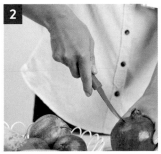
Cut hole in top with knife.

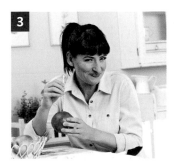
Insert straw and enjoy!

Herb of Immortality Tea

Jiaogulan, also known as herb of immortality, is said to have rejuvenating properties. Studies from Asia confirm that, indeed, the herb has powers resembling those of ginseng. However, it is significantly better at fortifying the immune system, lowering blood pressure and supplying antioxidants.

When to Use It

For revitalizing and rejuvenating.

How to Use It

To get the full benefit from this tea, drink two cups a day; tea lovers can drink more if they like. Herb of immortality does not have a stimulating effect, so you can drink it in the evening before going to bed.

You Will Need

- Sharp knife
- Cutting board
- Tea strainer
- 2 teacups
- Fine-mesh sieve

7 to 10	fresh herb of immortality shoots (or 1 tsp/5 mL dried herb of immortality leaves)	7 to 10
	Liquid honey or lemon juice (optional)	

How to Make It

1. Using a sharp knife and a cutting board, finely chop fresh herb of immortality shoots. If using dried leaves, pick leaves off stems. Place shoots in a tea strainer inside a teacup.

2. Pour boiling water over top. Cover and let steep for 5 minutes so that the tea can develop its full effect. Don't let leaves steep for much longer because the tea can turn bitter.

3. Strain the tea through a fine-mesh sieve into a second cup. If you like, sweeten the tea with a little honey, or add a dash of lemon juice.

Tips

Herb of immortality will happily grow on a windowsill or in a garden. It likes moisture but doesn't require a lot of care and is generally hardy in cool climates. Ask your local garden center whether they can order the plant for you, or search on the Internet for an online nursery that sells it (see Resources, page 246).

If you don't feel like dirtying a knife and a cutting board to make this tea, you can chop the herb of immortality shoots with a pair of sturdy kitchen shears.

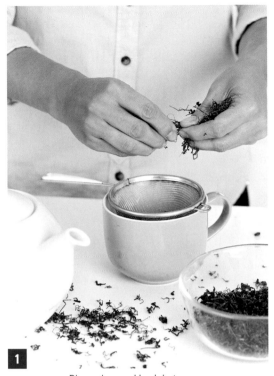

1 Place chopped herb in teacup.

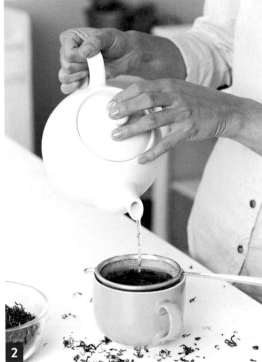

2 Pour boiling water over top.

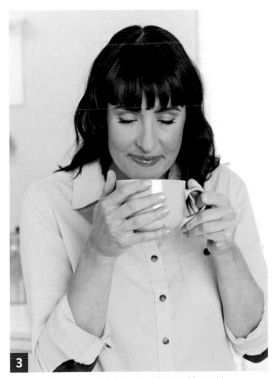

3 Enjoy tea, with honey or lemon if you like.

Everything Else You Might Need

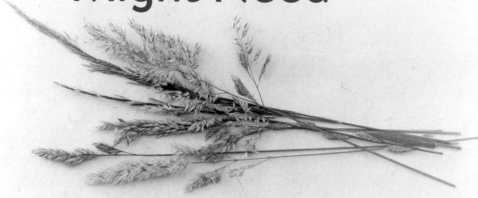

OK, be honest: Are you one of the great majority of people who spend the day seated (without getting any exercise in your scarce leisure time)? Do you top it all off by not eating a balanced diet? Don't worry—I won't bore you by repeating the usual advice about getting to the root of the problem before doing permanent damage to your health. I'll restrict myself to offering up a few remedies that will help you deal with the consequences of a comfortable lifestyle.

An Ounce of Prevention Is Worth a Pound of Cure

We all know that, in the long term, mere "damage control" is not good enough. Make a resolution, therefore, to cold-shoulder elevators and escalators starting tomorrow. For the next week, take two steps at a time when you climb the stairs, and walk once around the block in the evening. At some point, probably fairly soon, you'll completely banish your weaker self and find yourself going for a jog in the park twice a week.

My Favorite Recipes for All Sorts of Complaints

In the next few pages, you'll find my first lines of defense against digestive problems, backaches and more. If you're trying to find a remedy to treat hemorrhoids, head back to Yarrow Balm (page 120). For a heartburn-busting recipe, check out Healing Vinegar (page 85).

Fig Syrup (page 142)

You probably already know that dried figs are a great remedy for constipation. But I actually much prefer taking a syrup made from fresh figs. The effect is the same, perhaps even a little better thanks to the added psyllium seeds (see page 148 for another way to use them).

Anti–Cold Sore Balm (page 144)

When a cold sore rears its ugly head, I always advise my patients to dab a bit of honey onto the affected area. In my experience, honey makes cold sores disappear quickly and hurt less because it kills bacteria and disinfects. Cold sores, caused by a type of herpes virus, can be treated even more successfully with lemon balm. Studies have shown that its antiviral action starts to take effect after only a few hours. If you tend to suffer from cold sores, keep a supply of this cream ready at home.

Tea Tree Oil Mouthwash (page 145)

Contrary to popular belief, bad breath is not caused by a sick stomach. In about 90% of all cases, halitosis originates in the oral cavity or in the nose and throat, where smelly sulfur and nitrogen compounds are formed by decomposing food particles. That means most cases of bad breath are not a big health concern. But bad breath will ensure that others keep their distance. This tea tree oil mouthwash will quickly make you socially acceptable again.

Bitters (page 146)

After a rich meal, nothing helps digestion better than a sip of homemade bitters. The bitter constituents in the medicinal herbs that I've selected stimulate the production of saliva, gastric juices and bile, all of which are conducive to good digestion. By the way, presented in an attractive small bottle, these bitters make an excellent present for the host when you're invited to share a meal with friends.

Psyllium (Fleawort) Seeds (page 148)

These seeds with the funny name swell in the stomach, making them a popular remedy (in combination with diet) to curb hunger. In addition, in the 1990s, it was proven that psyllium seeds lower cholesterol levels. That has made them a widely used nutritional supplement, especially in the United States. Researchers are currently studying whether the seeds are also able to lower elevated blood sugar levels. In my opinion, there are few remedies better able to encourage sluggish bowels than psyllium.

Moringa Smoothie (page 149)

Make sure you check out how unbelievably healthy moringa is on page 206. I don't want to bore you with numbers, but they're impressive. A 3.5-oz (100 g) portion of moringa leaves contains seven times more vitamin C than oranges, four times more vitamin A than carrots, four times more calcium than milk, three times more potassium than bananas and twice as much protein as soybeans. The most astonishing property of moringa seeds is that they can purify polluted water. Swiss researchers have discovered that just 0.007 oz (0.2 g) of pulverized moringa seeds are needed to turn 4 cups (1 L) of polluted water into potable water. In Africa, moringa is used in many places for water treatment. I, however, use moringa powder to mix up this delicious smoothie. If you drink it every day, there's no need for expensive vitamin pills.

Hay Bag (page 150)

For tension, and back or joint aches, I like to prescribe a warm hay bag. Its combination of humidity and heat quickly makes muscles supple. This little bag also stimulates blood flow to the liver, thereby detoxifying the entire body and helping cells regenerate. To stimulate the liver, simply place the warm bag on the upper right quadrant of the abdomen, hold it in place with a thick cotton cloth and lie on the couch for half an hour. It's a cozy, relaxing treatment.

Fig Syrup

Millions of people around the world regularly complain about constipation. When it is acute, this fig syrup will quickly get your bowels back into the swing of things. High-fiber senna leaves stimulate intestinal motility, while psyllium seeds swell and soften the stool, promoting elimination.

When to Use It

For constipation.

How to Use It

Take 1 to 2 tsp (5 to 10 mL) syrup per day with plenty of fluids, preferably after the evening meal.

Shelf Life

The syrup will keep for about 3 weeks in the fridge.

Caution

Don't take this syrup for more than 2 or 3 days in a row, because prolonged use of senna can irritate the mucous lining of the intestines. Do not use this syrup if you have inflammatory bowel disease—the inflamed intestines should not be stimulated further.

You Will Need

- Tea strainer
- Teacup
- Sharp knife
- Cutting board
- Blender (or immersion blender and tall container)
- Small saucepan
- Wooden spoon
- Dark bottle (8 oz/250 mL)

0.5 oz	dried senna leaves	15 g
8	fresh figs	8
1	piece (¾ inch/2 cm long) fresh ginger	1
3.5 oz	granulated sugar	100 g
1 tbsp	psyllium seeds	15 mL
	Juice of 1 lemon	

How to Make It

1. Place senna leaves in a tea strainer inside a teacup. Pour 7 tbsp (100 mL) boiling water over top and allow the leaves to swell for a few minutes. Squeeze out the leaves and discard.

2. Briefly rinse figs under cold water. Using a sharp knife and a cutting board, quarter figs. Peel and very finely dice ginger.

3. In a blender, purée together figs, ginger, senna leaf tea and sugar. In a small saucepan, combine puréed mixture and psyllium seeds. Slowly heat mixture, stirring constantly with a wooden spoon, until syrupy. Stir in lemon juice.

4. Pour hot syrup into a dark bottle. Seal the bottle.

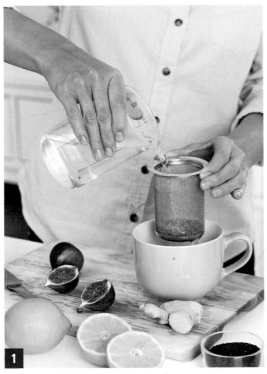

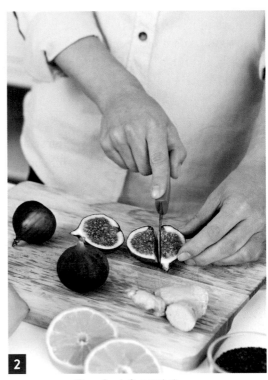

1 Prepare senna leaf tea.

2 Chop fresh figs and ginger.

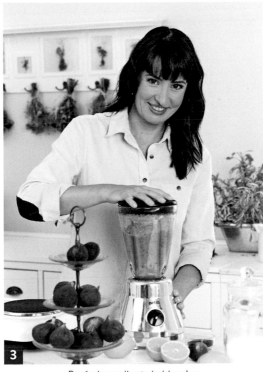

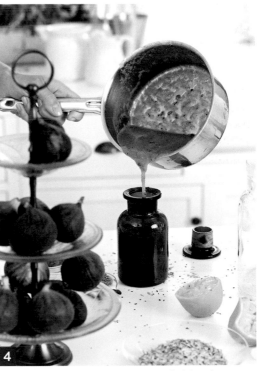

3 Purée ingredients in blender.

4 Heat mixture, then pour into dark bottle.

Anti–Cold Sore Balm

Lemon balm is extremely calming, which is why it's long been a trusted remedy for nervous problems, sleep disorders and minor gastrointestinal illnesses. It's a veritable virus slayer, making it a surefire weapon in the fight against cold sores.

When to Use It

For cold sores.

How to Use It

Dab a little of the balm onto cold sores several times a day. Wash your hands afterward to prevent spreading the virus.

Shelf Life

The balm will keep for about 6 months.

Tip

It takes 3 days to make this balm. If you frequently suffer from cold sores, it's a good idea to prepare some balm ahead of time so you're ready when the next outbreak hits.

You Will Need

- Sharp knife
- Cutting board
- Saucepan
- Cheesecloth or fine-mesh sieve
- Small lidded jars

| 2 | handfuls fresh lemon balm leaves | 2 |
| 8 oz | lard | 250 g |

How to Make It

1. Using a sharp knife and a cutting board, chop lemon balm leaves as finely as possible.

2. In a saucepan, melt lard. Stir in lemon balm. Simmer mixture gently for a few minutes. Take the saucepan off the heat, cover and set aside in a cool place for 3 days.

3. Reheat mixture until lard is melted again. Strain through cheesecloth into lidded jars. Let stand until set.

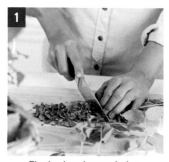
Finely chop lemon balm.

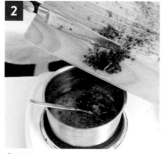
Stir lemon balm into melted lard.

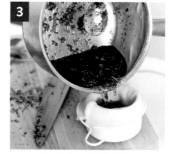
Strain into lidded jar.

Tea Tree Oil Mouthwash

Bacteria in the mouth and throat are often the cause of bad breath. The natural pharmacy offers a variety of effective medicinal plants to treat it. Tea tree, lavender and clove essential oils are a nearly unbeatable trio, full of active substances that ward off bacteria, fungi and inflammation.

When to Use It

For bad breath and inflamed gums.

How to Use It

Vigorously shake the bottle before every use. In the morning and evening, gargle and rinse with a sip of the mouthwash.

Shelf Life

The mouthwash will keep for about 2 weeks.

You Will Need

- Funnel
- Dark bottle (8 oz/250 mL)

1 cup	mineral water (still, not sparkling)	250 mL
2 tbsp	vodka	30 mL
6	drops tea tree essential oil	6
6	drops lavender essential oil	6
3	drops clove essential oil	3

How to Make It

1. Using a funnel, pour mineral water and vodka into a dark bottle.
2. Add tea tree, lavender and clove essential oils to the bottle.
3. Seal bottle and shake well to combine.

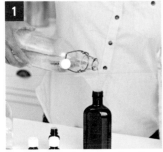
Pour mineral water and vodka into dark bottle.

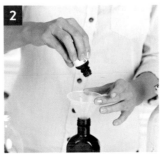
Add essential oils.

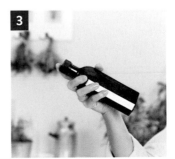
Shake to combine.

Bitters

The well-balanced mix of herbs in this bitter drink stimulates bile production and helps the digestive system break down fats. It also has antispasmodic and gas-fighting powers. In short, these bitters are a must-have for every household.

When to Use It

For improving and supporting digestion.

How to Use It

When needed, drink one liqueur glass of bitters after a meal.

Shelf Life

The bitters will keep for at least 1 year.

Tip

Don't fancy any alcohol? Then simply prepare a digestive tea. Place ½ tsp (2 mL) each dried wormwood leaves and dried rhubarb root in a teacup, pour a generous ¾ cup (200 mL) boiling water over top, cover and let steep for 10 minutes. Beware: The tea is very bitter because these digestion-stimulating substances contain bitter compounds.

You Will Need

- Large preserving jar (6 cups/1.5 L)
- Funnel
- Fine-mesh sieve
- Dark bottle (32 oz/1 L)

5 oz	dried centaury	150 g
3.5 oz	dried rhubarb root	100 g
3.5 oz	juniper berries	100 g
1.8 oz	dried yarrow leaves	50 g
1 oz	dried sweet flag root	30 g
0.7 oz	dried wormwood leaves	20 g
4 cups	vodka	1 L

How to Make It

1. Place centaury, rhubarb root, juniper berries, yarrow, sweet flag root and wormwood in a large preserving jar.

2. Pour vodka over herbs, roots and berries. Seal the jar and place it in a warm spot (preferably near a radiator or on a sunny windowsill) for 2 weeks. At regular intervals, vigorously shake the jar.

3. Using a funnel and a fine-mesh sieve, strain the liquid into a dark bottle. Seal bottle.

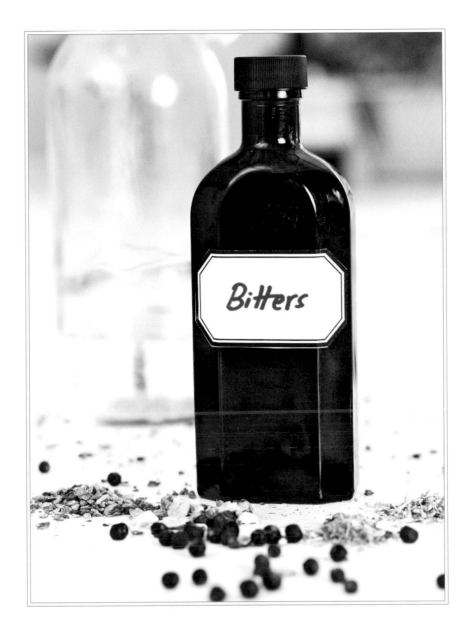

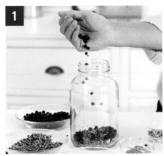

1

Place herbs, berries and roots in preserving jar.

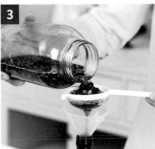

2

Pour vodka over top.

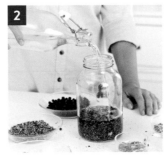

3

Strain into bottle.

Psyllium (Fleawort) Seeds

The seeds of a medicinal plant traditionally called fleawort (that, luckily, has no connection with fleas), psyllium seeds are increasingly popular. They swell markedly in the stomach, which naturally reduces appetite and helps with weight loss. And all this without habituation or the side effects of conventional diet aids.

When to Use It

For weight loss (to complement and support a diet) and for sluggish bowels.

How to Use It

Start with a small dose of 1 tsp (5 mL) twice a day (that's about 0.35 oz/10 g). Slowly increase to 4 tsp (20 mL) twice a day (that's equal to the maximum dose of 1.4 oz/40 g). How you feel will determine the correct dosage for you.

Shelf Life

The psyllium seeds will keep for at least 1 year.

You Will Need

Psyllium seeds or psyllium seed husks (not ground)

How to Make It

1. Take 1 tsp (5 mL) psyllium seeds with a glass of water twice a day, drinking plenty of liquid between doses. Do not soak the psyllium seeds before taking them; this would prevent them from swelling in the stomach.

Tip

In order for psyllium seeds to swell in the stomach, you must drink plenty of liquid—ideally 6 to 8 cups (1.5 to 2 L) per day. The best choices are water, unsweetened herb and fruit teas, or heavily diluted fruit juice. Milk is not suitable, because it hinders the swelling of the seeds.

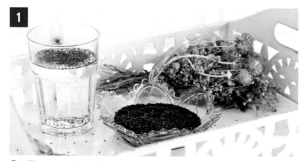

Psyllium seeds and fresh water make a great weight loss team.

Moringa Smoothie

Want to give your body optimum care, but don't want to swallow a lot of powders, pills and other medicines every day? If you want to look and feel healthy, this is the recipe for you. Moringa is one of the most nutritious plants in the world.

When to Use It

For improving general well-being.

How to Use It

Drink one smoothie each day. (Personally, I don't like eating breakfast, so I get a healthy start to my day with this energy drink.) Take a 4-week break after 3 months to avoid getting habituated.

Shelf Life

This smoothie doesn't keep; always blend a fresh one to ensure maximum vitamin content.

You Will Need

- Blender
- Large glass
- Straw

2 tbsp	dried goji berries	30 mL
7 tbsp	pomegranate juice (see tips, below)	100 mL
7 tbsp	soy milk or full-fat milk	100 mL
2 tbsp	flaxseeds	30 mL
2 tsp	moringa leaf powder (rounded teaspoonfuls)	10 mL
1 or 2	ice cubes	1 or 2

How to Make It

1. Spoon goji berries into a blender.
2. Add pomegranate juice, soy milk, flaxseeds, moringa powder and ice cubes. Blend at high speed for 10 seconds or until well combined.
3. Pour smoothie into a large glass, add a straw and enjoy this natural source of vitality immediately.

Tips

Commercial pomegranate juice often has additives. For the best nutrition in this smoothie, freshly press your own juice (see page 137) or choose a bottle labeled "100% juice."

Spooning the goji berries into the blender before adding the liquid ensures the blades will chop them finely.

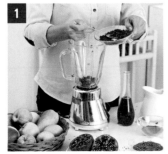
Spoon goji berries into blender.

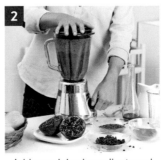
Add remaining ingredients and blend well.

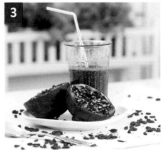
Enjoy immediately.

Hay Bag

A hot hay bag is a traditional remedy for aches of the locomotive system (your muscles and bones). It stimulates metabolism and increases blood flow, allowing muscles to relax. People who are allergic to pollen can usually tolerate this treatment, because little pollen escapes the bag and reaches the respiratory tract.

When to Use It

For back pain, muscle tension and aching joints.

How to Use It

Carefully test the temperature of the bag on the inside of your wrist. When it's comfortable to the touch, place the bag on the aching body part (you can use a blanket or towel in addition to the bag). If possible, rest for 30 to 40 minutes with the bag on. Take the bag off once it has cooled down or no longer feels pleasant.

Shelf Life

You can reuse the filled hay bag up to three times.

Tip

Look for fresh hay and hay flowers at organic stores. If you're lucky enough to live near a farm that raises hay, ask the farmer for a few handfuls.

You Will Need

- Cotton bag (or small zippered pillowcase)
- Ribbon or string
- Steamer basket or sieve
- Large pot
- Kitchen tongs

| 2 | handfuls fresh hay and hay flowers (see tip, at left) | 2 |

How to Make It

1. Fill a cotton bag with hay and flowers and tie closed with a ribbon. (Alternatively, put the hay into a small pillowcase and zip closed.)

2. Lightly sprinkle bag with cold water.

3. Insert a steamer basket into a large pot. Fill with just enough boiling water to come up under steamer basket without touching it. Place hay bag into steamer basket and steam for about 20 minutes. Caution: Do not let the bag touch the water directly. Using kitchen tongs, remove hot bag from pot.

4. Let bag cool enough to handle. Carefully test the bag temperature on the inside of your wrist to ensure it's comfortable to use.

Caution

Never place a hay bag on an open wound (it hurts!). Don't use the bag for acute, inflamed infections or to treat high fevers—the added heat is totally counterproductive for the body.

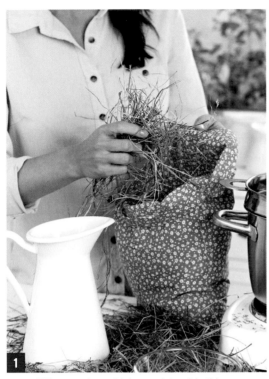

Fill cotton bag with hay and tie with ribbon.

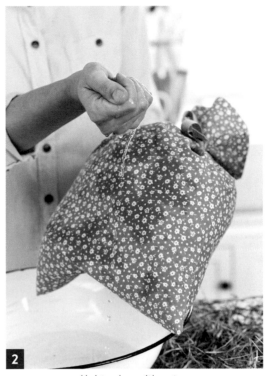

Moisten bag with water.

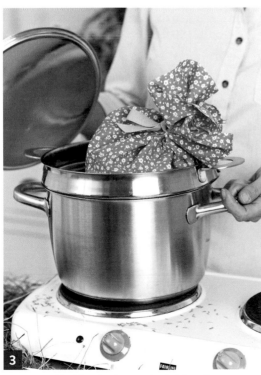

Heat bag in steamer basket in pot.

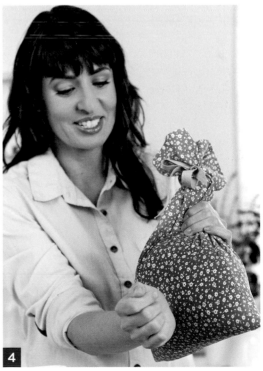

Carefully check temperature before use.

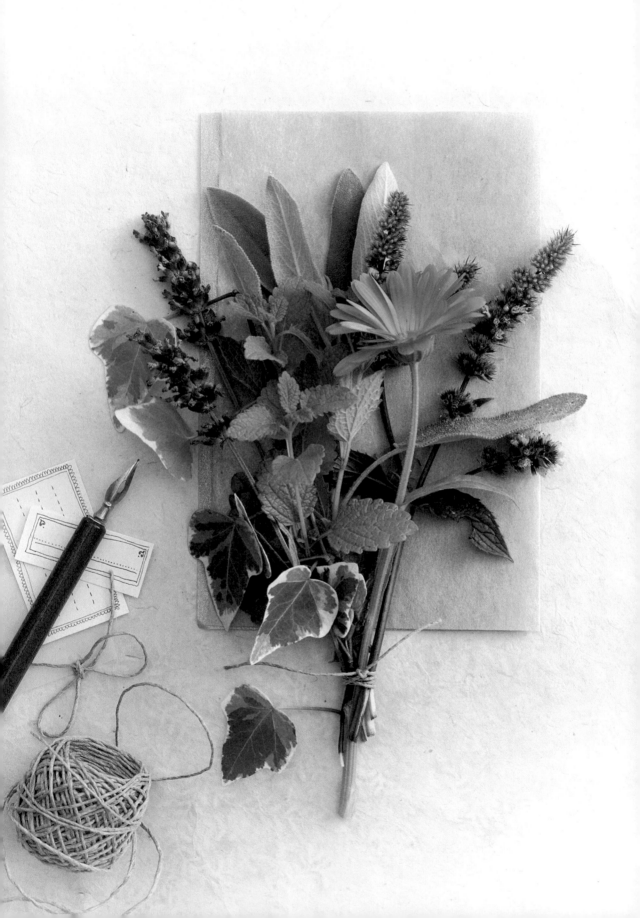

The Most Important Medicinal Plants

So you'd like to read some more about medicinal plants? Of course! On the following pages you'll find, in alphabetical order, all the essential information about the 81 plants I used to create the recipes in this book. Many of these plants are used in age-old home remedies, but there are also a few unexpected "exotics" among them that have quite a lot of potential for health enhancement.

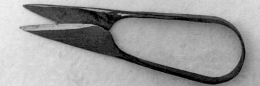

Plant Portraits from A–Z

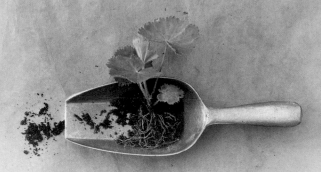

Unfortunately, it's not possible—yet—to capture the superb aroma of medicinal plants between the covers of a book. But at least I can tell you about Mother Nature's "medicinal sledgehammers," and show you, in photographs, that many of these plants are also really beautiful to look at. I hope that after you browse through this small encyclopedia of medicinal plants, herbal medicine will have won your heart, too.

Plant Profiles

The individual plant portraits in this chapter are all structured in the same way, using the same headings:
- Names (English and Botanical)
- Where Does It Grow?
- What Does It Look Like?
- Which Parts Are Used?
- What Does It Do?
- How Can I Use It?
- What Do Scientists Think of It?
- Caution

English Names
These are the common English names used in North America for the plants. I use these names in the recipe section of the book.

Botanical Names
Many traditional medicinal herbs have a number of different common names, and some vary according to region. To prevent any confusion, it is therefore useful to list the correct scientific name, or botanical designation, for each medicinal plant under the English name. This Latin name usually has two parts: the first indicates the genus; the second, the species. This binomial nomenclature system was developed by the Swedish botanist Carolus Linnaeus (a.k.a. Carl von Linné or Carl Linnaeus), whom I mentioned earlier (see page 13).

Where Does It Grow?
Here, you'll find out in which part of the globe the medicinal plant originated, as well as where it is being cultivated today.

What Does It Look Like?
Under this heading, I describe the most important external features of each plant; for example: How tall does it grow? What do the leaves look like? When does it flower? What color are the flowers?

Which Parts Are Used?
Medicinal plants usually contain several substances that are medicinally active. How much of a substance a plant contains

depends on where it grows, the weather, the time of harvesting and the way it is processed. In addition, different parts of the plant also contain different amounts of active substances.

Under this heading, you'll learn which parts of a plant are normally used, because experience or scientific studies have shown that they contain the highest levels of medicinally active components.

What Does It Do?

Under this heading, you'll find out which health complaints a plant was traditionally used to treat. You'll also find out for what purposes it is mainly used today.

How Can I Use It?

This is the practical part. Here, you'll find references to the recipes in this book that use that particular plant. If the plant is also suitable for other quick preparations (mostly teas), I've also added that information under this heading.

What Do Scientists Think of It?

Very briefly, in this section, I have included information on whether the plant has been scientifically endorsed in studies or by specific regulatory bodies. See the Scientific Endorsements box, below.

Caution

If you need to watch out for contraindications while making a remedy or using a particular medicinal plant (for example, because it should not be given to pregnant women or people suffering from certain diseases), you'll find out about it under this heading.

Scientific Endorsements
· ·

Different countries have different standards for herbs and plant-based medicines. Check with national and state or provincial governments to verify local information, regulations and recommendations for use. In North America, look for information from the Food and Drug Administration (FDA) or the National Center for Complementary and Alternative Medicine (NCCAM). In Canada, check with Health Canada about natural medicines and supplements.

In Europe, plant-based medicines are widely researched and regulated. Commission E is an independent scientific commission of experts at the German Federal Institute for Drugs and Medical Devices. The aim of the commission is to publish scientific and experiential material on the desired and undesired effects of plant-based drugs. The commission's members are appointed every three years. They are experts from the fields of biology, biometry, conventional medicine, natural medicine, pharmacology and toxicology.

ESCOP stands for European Scientific Cooperative on Phytotherapy, the name of a commission that works in a similar way to Commission E but at the European Union level. Information released by ESCOP is more up-to-date and comprehensive than that from Commission E, so it is more highly rated. You'll see both Commission E and ESCOP mentioned often in the following plant profiles under the What Do Scientists Think of It? heading.

Anise (Aniseed)

Pimpinella anisum

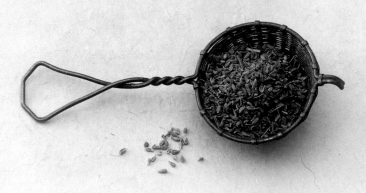

Where Does It Grow?

Originally a native of the Far East, anise also grows in Europe today.

What Does It Look Like?

An herbaceous annual plant that grows up to about 20 inches (50 cm) tall, with feathered leaves. The white, umbel-shaped flower clusters appear from June to September. The ripe seeds are harvested starting in August.

Which Parts Are Used?

The dried seeds and essential oil.

What Does It Do?

Mildly spicy, slightly sweet aniseed was already in use as a remedy in ancient Egypt. Today, it is mostly used for stomach or bowel complaints; for example, flatulence or colic-like pains. But it is also used for diseases of the respiratory tract, such as bronchitis and coughs. Aniseeed stimulates milk production in breastfeeding women, and, thanks to its antispasmodic properties, also helps alleviate menstrual cramps.

How Can I Use It?

Anti-Colic Tea (page 40), Expectorant Tea (page 75) and Breastfeeding Tea (page 119).

What Do Scientists Think of It?

The German Commission E and the European agency ESCOP (see page 155) endorse anise for the treatment of gastrointestinal conditions as well as for bronchitis and throat inflammations.

Caution

In rare cases, anise may cause allergic reactions of the skin, air passages or gastrointestinal tract.

Bearberry

Arctostaphylos uva-ursi

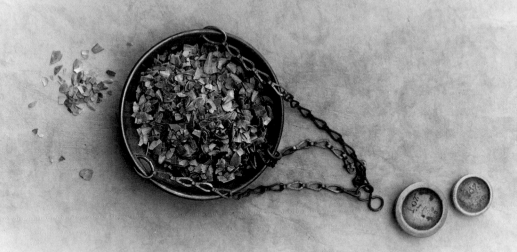

Where Does It Grow?
Europe, Asia and North America.

What Does It Look Like?
This evergreen groundcover plant has reddish-brown stems and leathery foliage. Small, white flowers appear from March to June and develop into pea-size scarlet berries. The plant is protected in Germany.

Which Parts Are Used?
The leaves.

What Does It Do?
Bearberry contains tannins and the active substance arbutin, which act as a diuretic, so the leaves are traditionally used for complaints of the urogenital tract, such as cystitis or urethritis. It is most effective when the urine is alkaline, so, during treatment, avoid eating meat, fish and dairy products.

How Can I Use It?
Bearberry Leaf Tea (page 103).

What Do Scientists Think of It?
Scientific studies have only been conducted on products that contain a mixture of bearberry leaves and other extracts, such as dandelion root. These preparations have proved successful for more than 1,000 urinary tract complaints.

Both the German Commission E and the European agency ESCOP (see page 155) endorse treatment with bearberry leaves for urinary tract infections as long as no antibiotics are required. If it is advisable to use an antibiotic, its effects are markedly increased when taken concurrently with bearberry leaves, thus speeding up the healing process.

Caution
Bearberry Leaf Tea (page 103) is not suitable for pregnant or breastfeeding women, or for children under the age of 12 years. In addition, medicines that contain arbutin must not be taken for longer than a week—and not exceeding five weeks in a year—as they can cause liver damage.

Because bearberry is high in tannins, sensitive patients may experience nausea and vomiting when using the plant. If the daily dosage of 0.35 oz (10 grams) is exceeded, bearberry may cause constipation.

Black Cohosh

Cimicifuga racemosa or *Actaea racemosa*

Where Does It Grow?
Originally in the forests of Canada and the United States; more recently, also cultivated in Europe.

What Does It Look Like?
This perennial plant, a member of the buttercup family, grows up to 8 feet (2.5 m) tall. From the frost-hardy, heavily branched, blackish rootstock grows an upright, smooth stem with large, triple-pinnate leaves. The large flower racemes consist of numerous small, whitish silver individual florets and appear in their full glory between June and September.

Which Parts Are Used?
The dried roots and rhizomes.

What Does It Do?
North America's indigenous peoples used black cohosh to treat rheumatism, sciatica and snake bites. Today, the plant has established a solid role in gynecological treatments. Black cohosh is used successfully to treat both menstrual cramps and typical complaints of menopause, because the active substances contained in its rootstock have a similar effect to that of the female sex hormone estrogen. While the two have very different chemical structures, the active compounds in black cohosh alter some estrogen receptors in cells so that they develop estrogen-like reactions, but without the typical side effects of conventional estrogen treatment.

How Can I Use It?
Black Cohosh Tincture (page 108).

What Do Scientists Think of It?
There are numerous studies of black cohosh's effects on menopause symptoms, but I want to mention just one in this context. In 2003, researchers at the University of Basel, Switzerland, examined 152 women aged 42 to 60 years old who were suffering from menopausal complaints. Participants took a proprietary black cohosh preparation every day over a period of three months, in differing dosages. At the end of the trial phase, 70% of the complaints had been alleviated, regardless of the dose administered. The German Commission E (see page 155) recommends black cohosh for premenstrual syndrome (PMS), and menstrual and menopause complaints. The European agency ESCOP (see page 155) also recommends it as a treatment for nervous irritability and sleep problems.

Caution
Do not take black cohosh during pregnancy, because it can induce labor. Women with estrogen-dependent tumors, such as those found in certain breast or uterine cancers, should make absolutely certain to consult their doctors before taking this remedy. According to trials, black cohosh is more likely to have a protective effect against them, but treatment should only be undertaken with medical supervision.

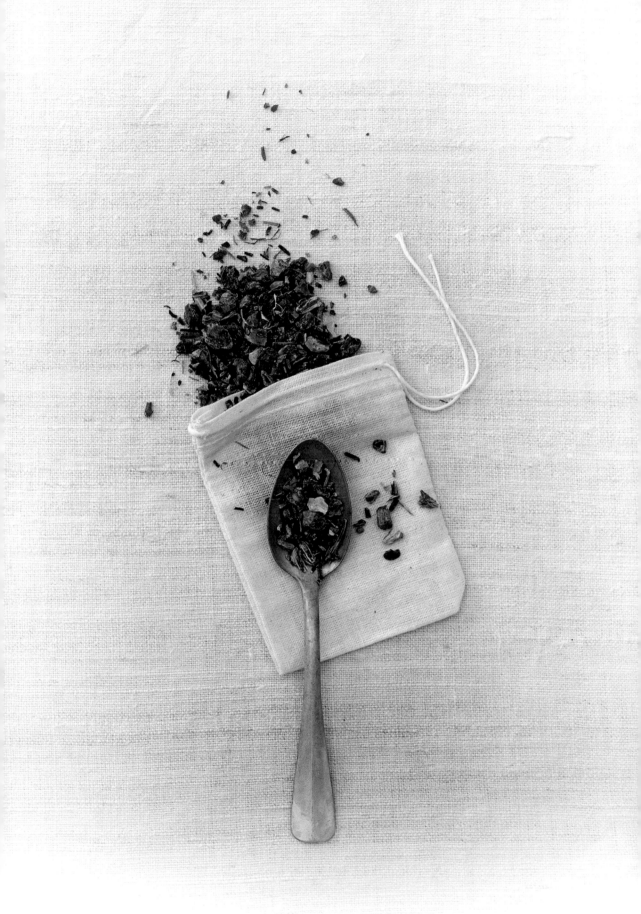

Caraway
Carum carvi

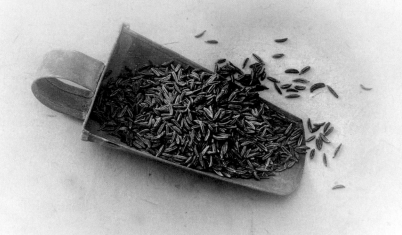

Where Does It Grow?
Wild in Europe, Asia and Africa; cultivated throughout the world.

What Does It Look Like?
This biennial herb has feathery leaves and white or pink flower clusters that appear from May to July. The aromatic, sickle-shaped brown seeds ripen between June and August.

Which Parts Are Used?
The seeds.

What Does It Do?
Caraway is one of the best medicinal plants for stomach and bowel complaints. Even for infants and young children, it alleviates flatulence and cramps in a gentle manner. In breastfeeding women, it stimulates milk production. Externally, caraway is used for rheumatic complaints, often as part of a compress (see page 25).

How Can I Use It?
Anti-Colic Tea (page 40) and Potato Decoction (page 114).

What Do Scientists Think of It?
Both the German Commission E and the European agency ESCOP (see page 155) recommend caraway seeds and oil for digestive complaints, flatulence, feelings of abdominal fullness and gastrointestinal pain.

Caution
If you are allergic to plants in the Asteraceae or Compositae (aster) family, or plants in the Apiaceae (carrot or parsley) family, you should not use caraway, because you risk an allergic reaction. There is no scientific evidence on the use of caraway during pregnancy or breastfeeding, so it is best to avoid the herb during these times.

Centaury

Centaurium erythraea

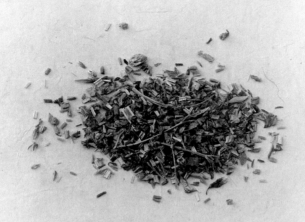

Where Does It Grow?
Europe, North Africa and North America.

What Does It Look Like?
This annual or biennial herb grows to almost 16 inches (40 cm) tall. The elongated oval leaves are arranged in rosettes at ground level and opposing on the stems. Between June and August, it forms pink flowers, which do not open until the temperature reaches 68°F (20°C).

Which Parts Are Used?
The entire flowering plant, except the root, is used.

What Does It Do?
Centaury is a member of the gentian family and, like its relatives, contains many bitter substances. It is used mainly for stomach and digestive tract complaints, to treat lack of appetite, and for liver and gallbladder problems. In phytotherapy, it is often combined with gentian.

How Can I Use It?
Healing Vinegar (page 85) and Bitters (page 146). To make a simple centaury tea, put 1 tsp (5 mL) dried centaury leaves into a cup, pour a generous $\frac{3}{4}$ cup (200 mL) boiling water over top, then cover and let steep for 10 minutes. The tea tastes very bitter; you're welcome to add some honey.

What Do Scientists Think of It?
There is, as yet, no compelling scientific evidence for the medicinal use of centaury, but the German Commission E (see page 155) endorses centaury for the treatment of digestive disorders and lack of appetite.

Caution
Do not use centaury if you are suffering from gastric, intestinal or duodenal ulcers. No other side effects are known.

Clove

Syzygium aromaticum

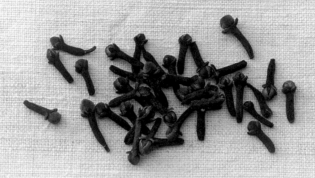

Where Does It Grow?

Originally in Indonesia; today, Zanzibar and Madagascar are the largest suppliers of cloves.

What Does It Look Like?

The flower buds of the small, evergreen clove tree first develop as yellowish-red flower clusters, then ripen into dark red berries. Like all parts of the tree, they are intensely aromatic and rich in essential oils.

Which Parts Are Used?

The unopened flower buds.

What Does It Do?

Clove essential oil, and especially its constituent substance, eugenol, have strong antibacterial and analgesic properties, and mild narcotic properties. This has firmly established the use of cloves in dentistry, where their oil is often employed to treat inflammation, pain and halitosis. Cloves also have a warming effect, stimulate digestion and help overcome nausea.

How Can I Use It?

Whole cloves in Clove Pack (page 41) and clove essential oil in Tea Tree Oil Mouthwash (page 145).

What Do Scientists Think of It?

The anti-inflammatory and antibacterial effects of cloves have been scientifically proven. The German Commission E (see page 155) therefore endorses their use for toothaches and inflammations of the mouth and throat.

Caution

Clove essential oil can easily cause skin irritation and should therefore not be used undiluted.

Comfrey

Symphytum officinale

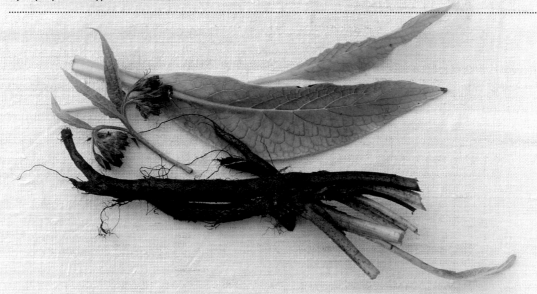

Where Does It Grow?
In moderate climatic zones all over Europe.

What Does It Look Like?
This perennial plant grows up to 4 feet (1.2 m) tall, with large, hairy and slightly wrinkled leaves. The yellowish-white, violet or crimson-colored bell-shaped flowers appear between the end of May and September. The roots are harvested in March and April, or October and November; the leaves are harvested in the summer.

Which Parts Are Used?
The leaves (fresh or dried), as well as the roots.

What Does It Do?
Comfrey kills pain, reduces swelling and assists in healing processes. People used comfrey in ancient times to treat bruises and broken bones—indeed, one of its popular names is "knitbone." Today, the plant is often used to treat sprains, backache, bursitis and sports injuries.

How Can I Use It?
Comfrey Ointment (page 54).

What Do Scientists Think of It?
A study of 143 patients with sprained ankle muscles demonstrated that, in at least two-thirds of participants, the use of comfrey ointment reduced the level of pain within eight days (in the control group that did not receive the ointment, less than one-third of patients enjoyed similar levels of pain relief). The German Commission E (see page 155) endorses the external use of comfrey for bruises, sprains and similar blunt-trauma injuries.

Caution
If used internally, large dosages of comfrey cause liver damage, so this form of treatment is not endorsed. Used externally, comfrey has no known side effects.

Common Ivy (English Ivy)

Hedera helix

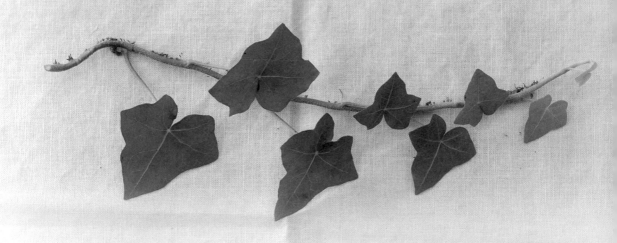

Where Does It Grow?
Western, central and southern Europe; southwestern Asia.

What Does It Look Like?
A woody groundcover plant or climber, common ivy has leathery, dark green and glossy evergreen leaves, with three to five lobes and light veins. The greenish yellow flower umbels appear from September to October.

Which Parts Are Used?
Mainly the leaves; rarely, the flowers.

What Does It Do?
Common ivy is used to treat respiratory problems, such as coughs (especially deep, chesty ones) and asthma (also known as spastic bronchitis). It is also taken for liver and gallbladder disorders, gout and rheumatism. It helps dilate airways, so it is a good supplementary treatment for obstructive bronchitis and asthma. The plant is used externally to cleanse wounds and as a cellulite remedy.

How Can I Use It?
Skin-Toning Oil (page 107).

What Do Scientists Think of It?
Both the German Commission E and the European agency ESCOP (see page 155) endorse the use of common ivy for inflammations of the air passages— especially in chronic bronchial diseases.

Caution
Fresh common ivy leaves and their sap may cause an allergic reaction on contact. Even ready-made preparations may lead to nausea and diarrhea. There are currently no scientific studies on the use of common ivy during pregnancy or breastfeeding; consult your physician or natural health practitioner before using it in those cases.

Coriander

Coriandrum sativum

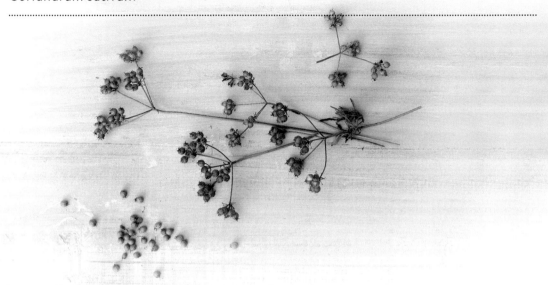

Where Does It Grow?
Originally East Asia; today, cultivated throughout the world.

What Does It Look Like?
Coriander is an annual herb that grows up to 2½ feet (80 cm) tall. The lower leaves are round to tripartite; the upper ones, finely divided and fern-like. White to pale red flower clusters appear from June to July; when fertilized, they become small, yellowish brown seeds up to ¼ inch (0.5 cm) in diameter.

Which Parts Are Used?
The seeds.

What Does It Do?
Coriander seeds stimulate appetite and digestion, and have an antispasmodic effect. They boost stomach activity and kill bacteria, and are therefore often included in preparations for gastrointestinal problems. Coriander's effect on these symptoms is, however, weaker than that of fennel (see page 170) and caraway (see page 160). In order to release their oils, coriander seeds must be crushed using a mortar and pestle before use; this also makes the seeds taste less bitter. Chewing coriander seeds helps fight bad breath. Coriander is also applied externally, as an ointment, for rheumatic complaints.

Tip
Coriander improves the taste of coffee and makes it easier to digest. Crush one or two seeds and stir them into your coffee.

How Can I Use It?
Anti-Colic Tea (page 40) and Love Liqueur (page 124).

What Do Scientists Think of It?
The German Commission E (see page 155) endorses coriander seeds and oil to treat lack of appetite and stomach disorders. In 2011, Portuguese researchers also tested the bactericidal action of coriander oil. The result: The oil was shown to kill 10 out of 12 bacterial strains, including the dreaded methicillin-resistant *Staphylococcus aureus* (MRSA) hospital germ and the food-borne strain of *Escherichia coli* (E. coli).

Cowslip

Primula veris

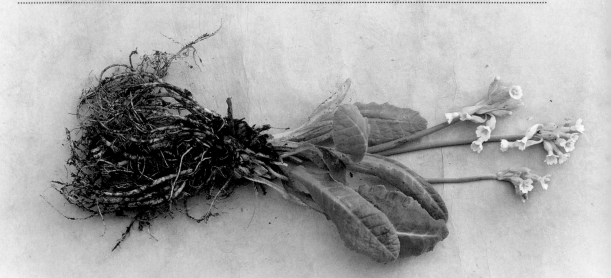

Where Does It Grow?
Primarily in Europe.

What Does It Look Like?
An herbaceous perennial plant, cowslip grows up to 8 inches (20 cm) tall, with a frost-hardy, short, thick root (rhizome). The oval leaves are arranged as a ground-hugging rosette; they are light green on the underside and dark green and wrinkly on top. The light yellow flower clusters bloom between March and April, exuding a pleasing, honey-like scent.

Which Parts Are Used?
The root and flowers.

What Does It Do?
Cowslip loosens phlegm and makes it easier to cough up. It also cleanses the blood and has a relaxing effect on the nervous system.

How Can I Use It?
Expectorant Tea (page 75) and Spring Tea (page 95).

What Do Scientists Think of It?
In 1999, the research group Monastic Medicine was founded at the University of Würzburg, Germany, with the aim of retrieving ancient knowledge about herbs and analyzing it scientifically in a contemporary context. Scientists in the group were able to demonstrate that cowslip loosens thick mucus when used to treat people suffering from a cough.

Caution
Cowslip plants are protected in the wild, and you are not allowed to collect them. For some people, skin contact with the flowers can lead to an itchy rash.

Dandelion

Taraxacum officinale

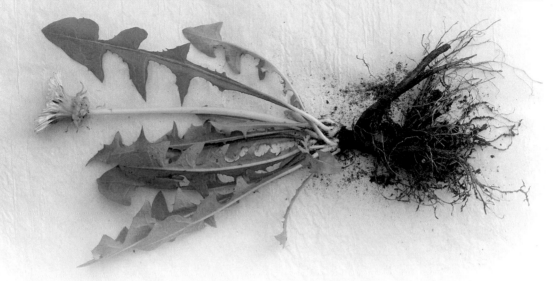

Where Does It Grow?
Central Europe; many different species grow across the globe.

What Does It Look Like?
The dandelion is a perennial composite plant that grows up to 12 inches (30 cm) tall, with unevenly lobed leaves and hollow stems. After blooming (from April to June), the golden yellow flowers turn into dandelion clocks, the puffy seedheads that children love to blow apart into the wind.

Which Parts Are Used?
The leaves, flowers and root.

What Does It Do?
Dandelion is known for its diuretic and detoxifying properties. It is often used to treat digestive disorders, abnormalities in liver or gallbladder function, gout and rheumatism.

How Can I Use It?
Spring Tea (page 95).

What Do Scientists Think of It?
Although there have been, as yet, no scientific trials on the use of dandelion, both the German Commission E and the European agency ESCOP (see page 155) recommend it for complaints of the gastrointestinal tract, for the restoration of liver and gallbladder function, and to boost urine flow.

Caution
Dandelion should not be used in the case of gallbladder or bowel obstruction. Consult your physician before using dandelion if you suffer from gallstones. Furthermore, contact with the milky sap exuded by the stems can cause allergic reactions in some people and can be toxic if ingested. The sap also leaves hard-to-remove stains on textiles.

Elderberry

Sambucus nigra

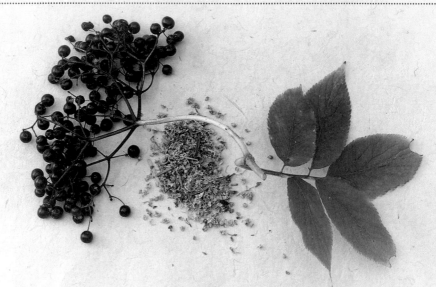

Where Does It Grow?
Europe.

What Does It Look Like?
A deciduous shrub or small tree that grows in hedges and on roadsides. Its bark is light gray and cracked, the leaves serrated. The strongly scented yellowish white flowers appear starting in May. The roughly ¼-inch (5 mm) diameter berries start to appear in August; they are red at first, then ripen to black. The juice is blood red and stains badly.

Which Parts Are Used?
Mainly the dried flowers, but the berries are used as well.

What Does It Do?
Both the flowers and the berries are antiviral and therefore helpful in treating colds with fevers, and flu-like infections. Elderberries are also considered to have anti-inflammatory and expectorant effects on bronchial infections and sinusitis. The berry juice is rich in vitamin C.

How Can I Use It?
Elderberry and Honey Syrup (page 44), Anti-Flu Tea (page 74) and Sinus Tea (page 77). The dried flowers can also be used alone to make a tea: put 1 tsp (5 mL) dried elder flowers in a cup and pour a generous ¾ cup (200 mL) boiling water over them; cover and let steep for 10 minutes.

What Do Scientists Think of It?
The German Commission E (see page 155) recommends elder flowers for colds. Studies conducted by Madeleine Mumcuoglu, an Israeli virologist, found that an elderberry extract is exceptionally successful at treating colds. It also hinders the proliferation of influenza viruses and considerably reduces the symptoms of flu.

Caution
Never use raw elderberries. The leaves, branches and bark of the elder tree are also slightly toxic.

Eyebright

Euphrasia officinalis

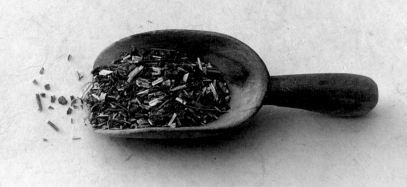

Where Does It Grow?
Europe.

What Does It Look Like?
Eyebright is an herbaceous annual plant that stands up to 12 inches (30 cm) tall; it has serrated leaves. The white, blue or reddish violet flowers, which have a conspicuous yellow spot on the three-lobed lower lip, appear from June to September; harvesting begins during the flowering season.

Which Parts Are Used?
The whole flowering herb.

What Does It Do?
Eyebright was used for eye disorders as early as the 14th century. It has anti-inflammatory, antispasmodic and antibacterial properties, which is why it is often used to treat conjunctivitis or inflammations of the eyelid margins. In popular medicine, eyebright was also taken internally as a tea to treat colds and coughs.

How Can I Use It?
Eyebright Compress (page 46).

What Do Scientists Think of It?
In 1986, the German Commission E (see page 155) found that there was too little evidence of the efficacy of eyebright and gave the use of the medicinal plant a negative rating for hygienic reasons. In the year 2000, however, an open-label clinical trial was conducted on the efficacy of eyebright drops in the treatment of conjunctivitis. The drops were well tolerated, and of the 65 study participants, 53 were cured completely after two weeks of treatment, and 11 others perceived a marked improvement in their condition.

Fennel

Foeniculum vulgare

Where Does It Grow?

A native of the Mediterranean region, fennel now grows in temperate zones almost anywhere in the world.

What Does It Look Like?

A highly aromatic perennial shrub that grows up to 8 feet (2.5 m) tall, with feathery leaves. The small yellow flower clusters appear from June to October; they develop into greenish, five-ribbed seeds.

Which Parts Are Used?

The seeds.

What Does It Do?

Fennel seeds are particularly rich in essential oils. These help relieve gas in infants and promote milk production in breastfeeding women. Thanks to its expectorant and antibiotic properties, fennel is often used for coughs. I also recommend a fennel steam bath for skin problems; it clears the complexion and makes pimples heal more quickly.

How Can I Use It?

Anti-Colic Tea (page 40), Fennel Honey (page 68), Irritable Cough Tea (page 76) and Breastfeeding Tea (page 119). To make a simple fennel tea, crush 1 tsp (5 mL) fennel seeds using a mortar and pestle and place in a cup. Pour boiling water over top, cover and let steep for 10 minutes. Strain and sip the tea slowly.

What Do Scientists Think of It?

The German Commission E (see page 155) recommends fennel for inflammatory diseases of the respiratory tract and for gastrointestinal tract complaints.

Caution

Unlike many other medicinal plants, which can be used more freely, fennel tea should only be consumed for a maximum of three weeks in a row. You should drink no more than five cups of fennel tea per day. Side effects can occur at higher doses.

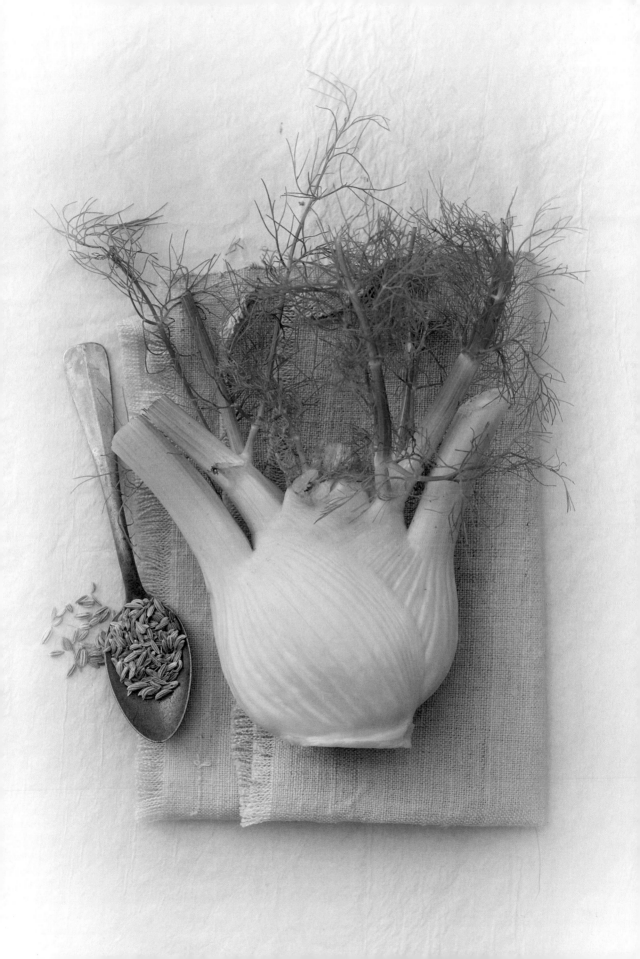

Fenugreek

Trigonella foenum-graecum

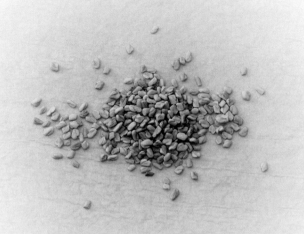

Where Does It Grow?

Mediterranean countries, Africa, India and Central Asia.

What Does It Look Like?

Fenugreek is an annual plant, between 4 and 20 inches (10 and 50 cm) tall, with widely branched stalks and an intense aroma. The leaves are reminiscent of clover. The pale yellow flowers are light violet at the lower ends and appear from April to July. They develop into husks, up to about 8 inches (20 cm) in length, that contain numerous pale yellow, cuboid seeds.

Which Parts Are Used?

The seeds.

What Does It Do?

Fenugreek contains many mucins, which calm the stomach and digestive tract, stimulate the appetite, and lower blood sugar and cholesterol levels. If applied externally, fenugreek makes boils and ulcers recede. In breastfeeding women, it stimulates lactation.

How Can I Use It?

Fenugreek Extract (page 89) and Breastfeeding Tea (page 119).

What Do Scientists Think of It?

Both the German Commission E and the European agency ESCOP (see page 155) recommend fenugreek internally to treat lack of appetite, and externally to treat local inflammations. ESCOP also recommends it for lowering blood sugar and cholesterol levels. In addition, a study in 2011 under the direction of Dr. Marion Moers-Carpi, a German dermatologist, demonstrated that fenugreek may be successfully used to prevent baldness by encouraging greater hair density and growth.

Caution

Too high a dose of fenugreek (3.5 oz/100 g a day or more) may cause stomach and bowel problems. In a few rare cases, people have suffered allergic reactions.

Fig

Ficus carica

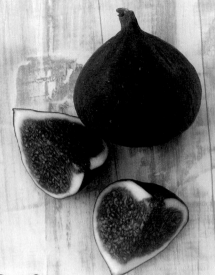

Where Does It Grow?

The fig tree is a native of the Middle East; today, it grows in many southern Mediterranean countries, but also in California and Australia.

What Does It Look Like?

A deciduous tree or shrub that grows 23 to 33 feet (7 to 10 m) tall, with conspicuous dark green, three- or five-lobed leaves that have soft, hairy undersides. The round to pear-shaped fruits are green- or dark violet–skinned, depending on the variety. The flesh of the fruit can be pale pink to purplish red, and is studded with numerous tiny edible seeds.

Which Parts Are Used?

The fruits.

What Does It Do?

Figs have anti-inflammatory properties, which is why, in the past, their flesh was applied to wounds. Today, the fig is better known as a mild laxative, because it contains plenty of fiber and potassium, thus speeding up the passage of waste through the digestive system. Thanks to the enzymes figs contain, they are also considered a tonic to fortify athletes, older people and anyone convalescing after a long illness. In popular medicine, the white sap exuded from the stem ends of the leaves is considered an excellent remedy for insect stings, because it alleviates itching.

How Can I Use It?

Fig Syrup (page 142).

What Do Scientists Think of It?

I am hoping that science will one day devote itself to studying this ancient medicinal fruit, but I have not been able to find any studies as yet.

Tip

Figs contain many minerals, such as calcium and magnesium, as well as vitamins B and C, and carotene. Although they taste delightfully sweet, each fruit contains only 30 to 40 calories. So, for your next sweet-tooth attack, try one of these fruits rather than chocolate.

Flaxseed (Linseed)

Linum usitatissimum

Where Does It Grow?
Around the world.

What Does It Look Like?
An annual, the flax plant has delicate stems and narrow, lance-shaped, gray-green leaves. It can reach a height of up to 5 feet (1.5 m). Short-lived, small, white-blue to blue flowers with a sky-blue style (the stalk connected to the stigma) appear between June and August. The flowers ripen into roundish seed capsules, each containing eight to 10 brown or black seeds.

Which Parts Are Used?
The seeds.

What Does It Do?
Flaxseeds are traditionally used as a natural digestive aid, thanks to their anti-inflammatory properties and the mucins they contain. Externally, flaxseeds are used in compresses to alleviate stomach pains and coughs.

Flaxseed oil is a vegetable oil with one of the highest concentrations of polyunsaturated fats. Its high levels of omega-3 fatty acids are also unique: 3.5 oz (100 g) flaxseed oil contains 55 g of omega-3 fatty acids (in comparison, 3.5 oz/100 g of an oily fish like mackerel only contains 3 g of omega-3 fatty acids). These healthy omega-3 fatty acids protect the body from cardiovascular disease, and bring relief from inflammatory illnesses, such as rheumatism, and intestinal diseases.

How Can I Use It?
Winner's Breakfast (page 50), Potato Decoction (page 114) and Moringa Smoothie (page 149). To relieve constipation, take 1 to 2 tbsp (15 to 30 mL) freshly ground flaxseeds three times a day, with plenty of fluids.

What Do Scientists Think of It?
Both the German Commission E and the European agency ESCOP (see page 155) endorse flaxseeds for the treatment of constipation and inflammations of the gastrointestinal tract. Currently, the focus of research on flaxseed oil is on its positive effects on the brain. The oil can improve memory and concentration, brighten the mood and prevent hyperactivity. Its cholesterol-lowering properties are also the subject of many studies.

Caution
Flaxseeds should never be taken by people who have a bowel obstruction; people with intestinal inflammation should take flaxseeds only when they have been cooked and have swelled with liquid, such as in porridge. Adverse side effects of flaxseed oil are known only for a high overdose (more than 3.5 oz/100 g a day). Due to its high content of perishable omega-3 fatty acids, flaxseed oil has a very limited shelf life. After opening, store the bottle in the fridge and use it up promptly. The oil should not be heated, and works best in dishes that contain protein-rich foods, such as fresh cheeses (try quark or fromage frais) and plain yogurt.

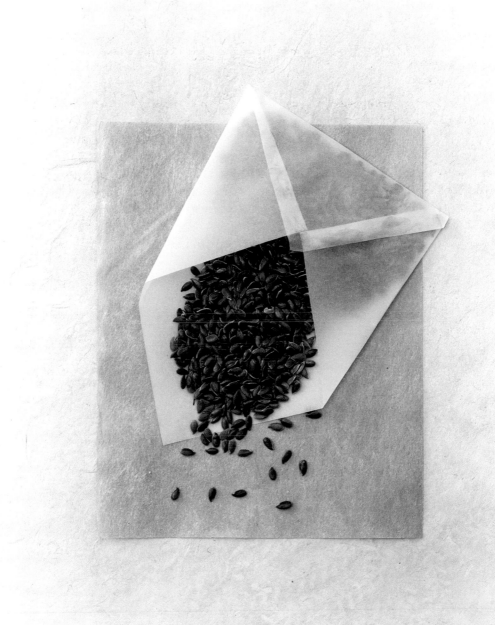

Garlic

Allium sativum L.

Where Does It Grow?
Probably originated in the Middle East and Mediterranean countries; today, garlic is cultivated around the world.

What Does It Look Like?
A member of the Allioideae subfamily of the Amaryllidaceae family, garlic has narrow, bluish-green leaves and white to pink flower heads that bloom in July and August. The bulb consists of a main clove and several subsidiary cloves, which are covered by a thin white or pinkish skin. As the flower dies off, the bulb thickens; it is harvested in late summer.

Which Parts Are Used?
The bulb.

What Does It Do?
The pungent garlic bulb kills bacteria and fungi, lowers blood pressure and cholesterol levels, dilates the blood vessels and improves blood flow. Garlic cleanses and calms the intestines, and, if taken regularly, is said to protect against heart attack and strokes.

How Can I Use It?
Garlic Drink (page 132). Chew some fresh parsley or basil after eating garlic to help banish bad breath.

What Do Scientists Think of It?
Both the German Commission E and the European agency ESCOP (see page 155) endorse garlic preparations for lowering high cholesterol levels and for preventing arteriosclerosis. ESCOP also recommends garlic to treat colds.

Caution
You shouldn't take any garlic preparations just before or after an operation, as they may affect blood coagulation.

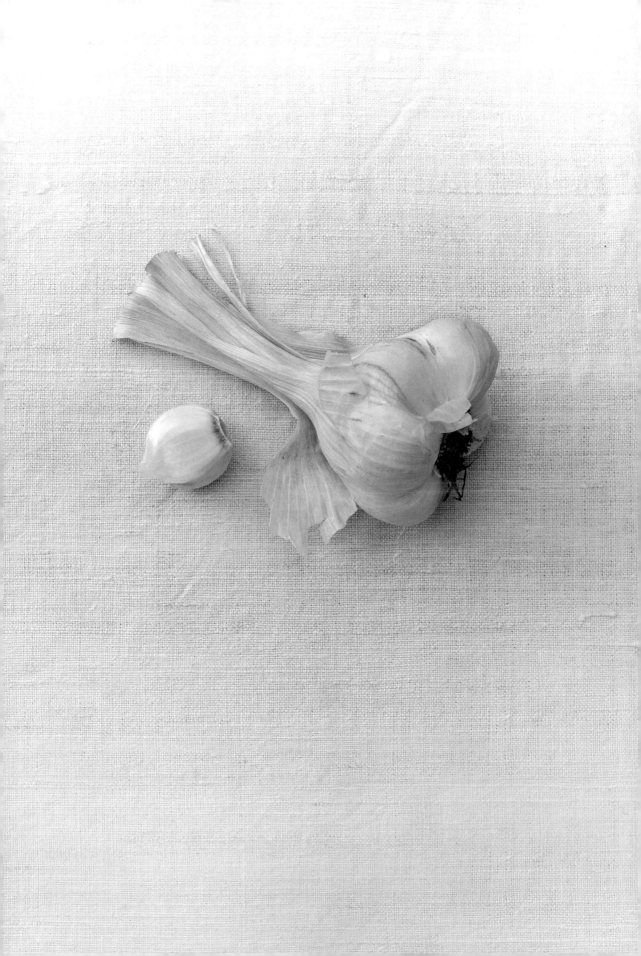

Ginger

Zingiber officinale

Where Does It Grow?

Originally from India and China; today, ginger grows in all tropical countries.

What Does It Look Like?

Ginger is a perennial, creeping plant, with reed-like stems that can reach more than 3 feet (1 m) in height; it has long, narrow leaves emerging from a bulbous rootstock (rhizome). The white to yellow flower clusters also rise directly from the rhizome.

Which Parts Are Used?

The rhizome.

What Does It Do?

In the past few years, ginger has steadily advanced from a culinary ingredient to a medicinal plant; even TV chefs emphasize the healing powers of this Asian rhizome. Perhaps best known is the power ginger exhibits in treating nausea, whether it's caused by motion sickness, morning sickness, chemotherapy or post-surgical recovery. Ginger has a warming effect on the body, so it also boosts the immune system. It is antibacterial, so it is an ideal companion during fall and winter, when colds abound. Ginger also brings relief for lack of appetite, nervous stomach complaints and flatulence.

How Can I Use It?

Ginger Candy (page 112), Rosemary Wine (page 134) and Fig Syrup (page 142). To treat colds (or prevent them), I recommend hot ginger water. Cut off a $\frac{3}{4}$-inch (2 cm) long piece of ginger, then peel and slice it. Place it in a cup, pour boiling water over top and let steep for 10 minutes. You can reuse these ginger slices to make many cups of tea.

What Do Scientists Think of It?

Both the German Commission E and the European agency ESCOP (see page 155) endorse ginger to prevent motion sickness and vomiting after minor operations, and to treat stomach and bowel complaints. In animal trials, ginger was demonstrated to have positive effects on arteriosclerosis and treating excessive weight gain.

Caution

Older herbal handbooks may say to avoid using ginger during pregnancy, but the most recent studies do not support this concern. On the contrary, ginger is very well suited to treating morning sickness. You should, however, only use it in moderation. If you suffer from gallstones and/or take medication that inhibits blood clotting, consult your doctor before using ginger.

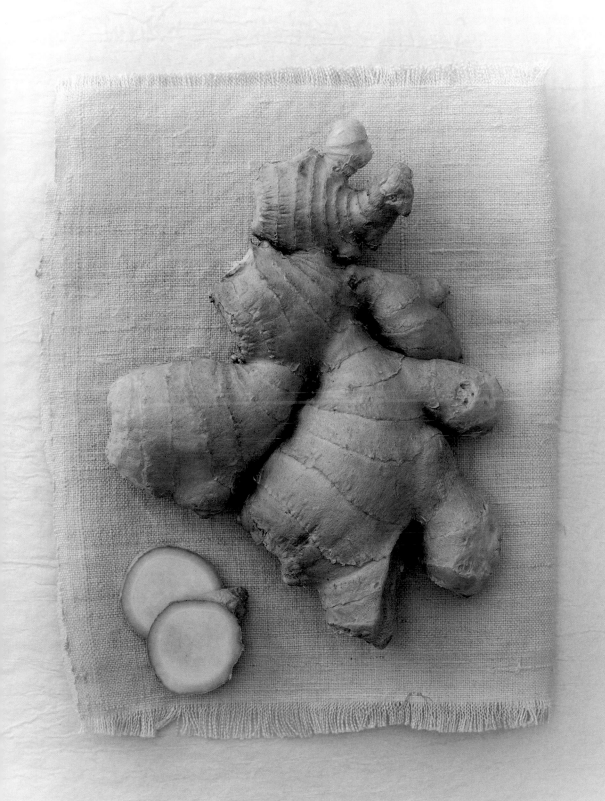

Goji Berry
Lycium barbarum

Where Does It Grow?
From southeastern Europe to China.

What Does It Look Like?
Goji berries are the fruits of the goji shrub, also known as the Chinese boxthorn, wolfberry or matrimony vine. This deciduous shrub with overhanging branches belongs to the Solanaceae family, and grows to $6\frac{1}{2}$ to 10 feet (2 to 3 m) tall. The attractive purple flowers bloom from June to September; they develop into fiery red, oval, $\frac{1}{2}$- to $\frac{3}{4}$-inch (1 to 2 cm) long fruits starting in August.

Which Parts Are Used?
The fruits.

What Does It Do?
In China, goji berries have been used for millennia to treat poor eyesight, and recently, the goji berry has become known in the media as a veritable panacea. It is said to strengthen the immune system, lower cholesterol levels, improve vision, lower blood pressure and slow the aging process. Although such hypotheses have not yet been scientifically proven, a look at the active ingredients in the berries confirms that it does, perhaps, have the qualities to qualify it as a superfruit. Goji berries contain 21 trace elements, 19 amino acids, more vitamin C than oranges and more carotenoids than any other food. Furthermore, they are rich in vitamin E, a situation that hardly ever occurs in fruits. Other substances in the fruit may help to increase the number of white blood cells, thus strengthening the immune system.

How Can I Use It?
Goji Berry Muffins (page 104) and Moringa Smoothie (page 149). Enjoy the muffins as a treat.

What Do Scientists Think of It?
Studies have demonstrated that the regular consumption of goji berries improves physical and mental performance, powers of concentration, well-being and quality of sleep. Goji berries also decrease stress and tiredness.

In addition, the polysaccharides contained in the berries are able to activate and encourage the multiplication of specialized immune cells called T-lymphocytes, which are, along with other cells, responsible for protecting the body against viruses and cancer.

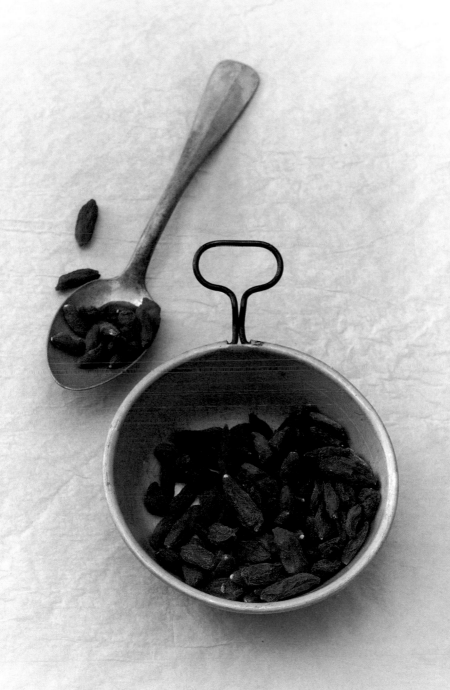

Greater Celandine

Chelidonium majus

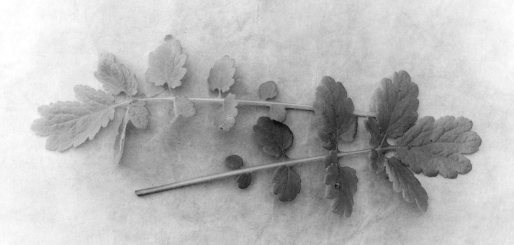

Where Does It Grow?
Europe and Asia.

What Does It Look Like?
This herbaceous perennial grows up to 28 inches (70 cm) tall, with gray-green, feathered leaves. Four-petaled yellow flowers appear from April to September.

Which Parts Are Used?
All parts that grow above-ground, which are collected and dried during the flowering period.

What Does It Do?
Greater celandine has been used since ancient times for the treatment of gallbladder and liver disorders, as well as for rheumatism and gout. Thanks to its antispasmodic effect, it is also used for menstrual cramps. It is used externally to treat skin diseases, such as eczema and warts.

How Can I Use It?
Skin-Toning Oil (page 107).

What Do Scientists Think of It?
Both the German Commission E and the European agency ESCOP (see page 155) recommend greater celandine for treating digestive disorders as well as cramp-like complaints in the upper abdomen and around the gallbladder and gall ducts.

Caution
Greater celandine should not be used internally by anyone with an obstruction in the gall ducts, by women who are pregnant or breastfeeding, or by children under 12 years of age. If you take a high-dosage ready-made celandine preparation for longer than four weeks in a row, you should have your liver enzymes checked. In rare cases, it can cause reduced liver function or jaundice. Once you stop using the remedy, these symptoms will completely disappear.

Ground Ivy

Glechoma hederacea

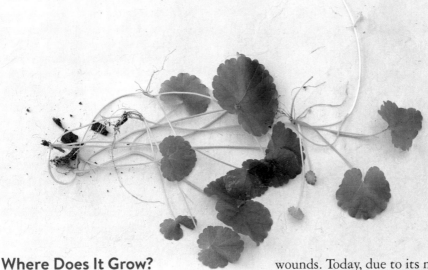

Where Does It Grow?
Europe and western Asia.

What Does It Look Like?
Ground ivy is an evergreen perennial, with heart or kidney-shaped leaves that have roughly notched edges. The undersides of the leaves are sometimes purple. The stems are densely covered in hairs, and the leaves may be as well. When rubbed between the fingers, the leaves exude a spicy aroma. The small blue-violet labiate flowers appear from May to June.

Which Parts Are Used?
The leaves.

What Does It Do?
Because of its astringent and anti-inflammatory properties, ground ivy was used as an external treatment for wounds that were healing badly, especially festering wounds. Today, due to its metabolism-boosting and astringent effects, the plant is often used externally to reduce fat in the body. It is also used internally for chronic, mucus-forming diseases of the respiratory tract.

How Can I Use It?
Skin-Toning Oil (page 107). You can also make a tea that's good for respiratory complaints or as a compress for badly healing or weeping wounds: put 1 tsp (5 mL) dried ground ivy leaves in a cup, pour a generous ¾ cup (200 mL) boiling water over top, cover and let steep for 10 minutes.

What Do Scientists Think of It?
Currently, no studies have been undertaken on using ground ivy as a medicinal plant, so there is a lack of scientific data.

Heartsease (Wild Pansy or Johnny-Jump-Up)

Viola tricolor

Where Does It Grow?

Flourishes in all temperate climate zones in Europe and Asia; also cultivated widely in North America as a decorative plant.

What Does It Look Like?

A perennial flowering plant of the violet family that grows to between 4 and 12 inches (10 and 30 cm) tall, with heart-shaped, elongated leaves. The flowers, which bloom from May to August, typically have three colors (hence the Latin name): blue-violet, yellow and white.

Which Parts Are Used?

The flowering plant.

What Does It Do?

Other pansy cultivars have virtually no healing powers, but the wild pansy is an excellent medicinal plant, especially for children, because it works very gently and is well tolerated. Heartsease is particularly good at bringing relief for the variety of skin diseases children experience, such as neurodermatitis, atopic eczema and diaper rash. It also relaxes the skin, alleviates pain and itching, and prevents infections. Heartsease is primarily used externally, but it can also be ingested in the form of tea (to treat colds and coughs, among other things).

How Can I Use It?

Heartsease Compress (page 47) and Spring Tea (page 95).

What Do Scientists Think of It?

The German Commission E (see page 155) recommends heartsease for minor weeping skin conditions as well as cradle cap. Generally, however, no significant studies of this plant have been undertaken.

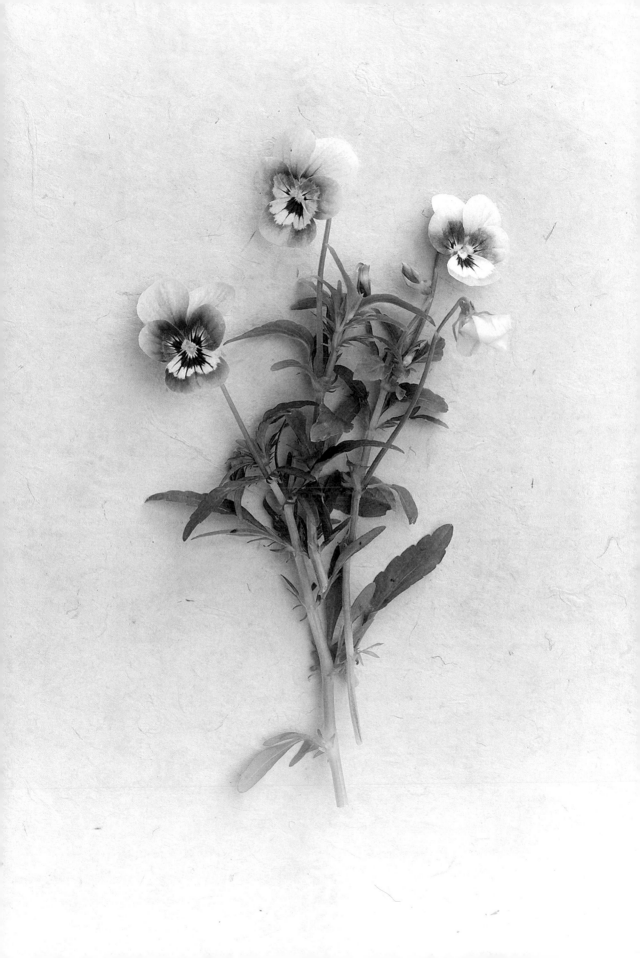

Herb of Immortality (Jiaogulan)

Gynostemma pentaphyllum

Where Does It Grow?
Asia.

What Does It Look Like?
This is an herbaceous climbing vine of the Cucurbitaceae family. The aboveground parts die off in winter but quickly proliferate again the following year, reaching a height of up to 26 feet (8 m). Small, greenish-white flowers appear from July to August, and turn into dark green to black, small, round berries after fertilization. This easy-care herb with five- to seven-fingered leaves is evergreen as a houseplant.

Which Parts Are Used?
The leaves; they can be harvested year-round and may be used fresh or dried.

What Does It Do?
The list of the plant's beneficial effects is long. Herb of immortality is said to regulate blood pressure and prevent heart attack and stroke by counteracting the clumping of blood platelets. It's also hemopoietic, which means it promotes the formation of blood cells. It contains tumor-inhibiting substances as well. Herb of immortality alleviates stress with its calming, harmonizing and regulating effects on the nervous system and, finally, promotes restorative sleep.

How Can I Use It?
Herb of Immortality Tea (page 138).

What Do Scientists Think of It?
A team of researchers from Japan became aware of herb of immortality during their search for alternative sweeteners more than 35 years ago. The foliage is sweet, so studies were carried out; they demonstrated that the herb boasted properties similar to those of ginseng, the eternally popular cure-all. In 1977, another team of Japanese scientists took up these studies and discovered that herb of immortality contains 82 different saponins—54 more than ginseng. These naturally occurring substances, which are present in various vegetables and other plants, bind to cholesterol in the gut, purge the body of toxins, improve elimination and inhibit the growth of tumors. Since then, much has been published about the active substances in and effects of herb of immortality. However, research is far from complete.

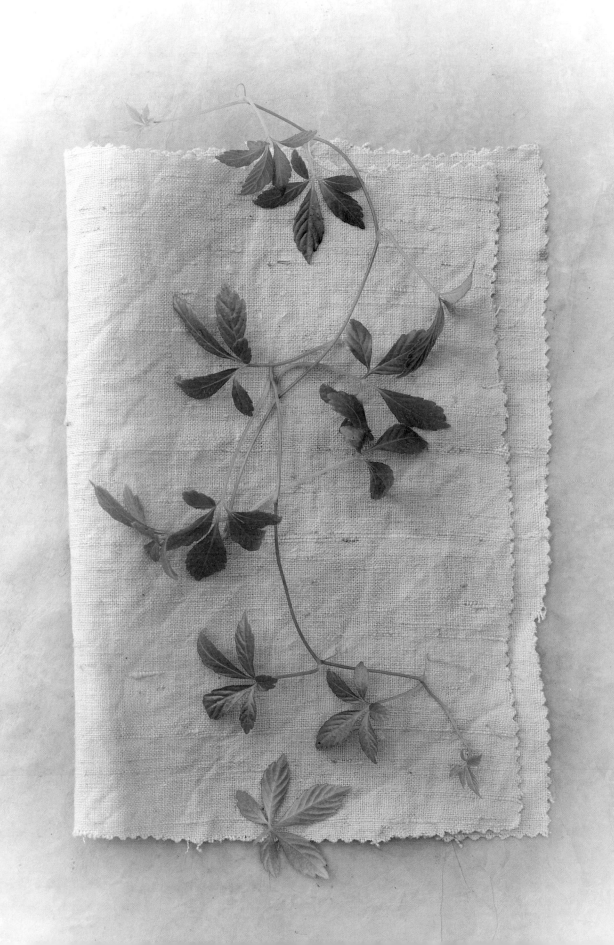

Holy Basil

Ocimum sanctum or *Ocimum tenuiflorum*

Where Does It Grow?
Asia and Australia.

What Does It Look Like?
An herbaceous perennial related to basil, woody around the base, holy basil grows up to 3 feet (1 m) tall. The elongated leaves and the branches are covered in fine hairs. The leaves are toothed along the margins and exude a pleasing aroma. Between June and September, the plant has white to purple flower spikes.

Which Parts Are Used?
The entire plant.

What Does It Do?
Holy basil, also known as Indian basil, is one of the most sacred plants for Hindus, and it plays an important role in Ayurvedic medicine. It has calming, relaxing, immunity-boosting, digestion-stimulating, antiseptic and cholesterol-lowering properties. Holy basil alleviates the symptoms of stress without making you feel tired. It calms the nerves and increases the powers of concentration.

How Can I Use It?
Anti-Stress Tea (page 88).

What Do Scientists Think of It?
In animal trials, clinical studies and laboratory studies, holy basil has been proven to kill bacteria, act as an analgesic and alleviate the symptoms of stress (among other effects, the plant lowers stress-induced hypertension). Recent studies are also examining whether the active substances in holy basil are capable of lowering elevated blood sugar levels.

Caution
Do not take holy basil if you are pregnant or breastfeeding.

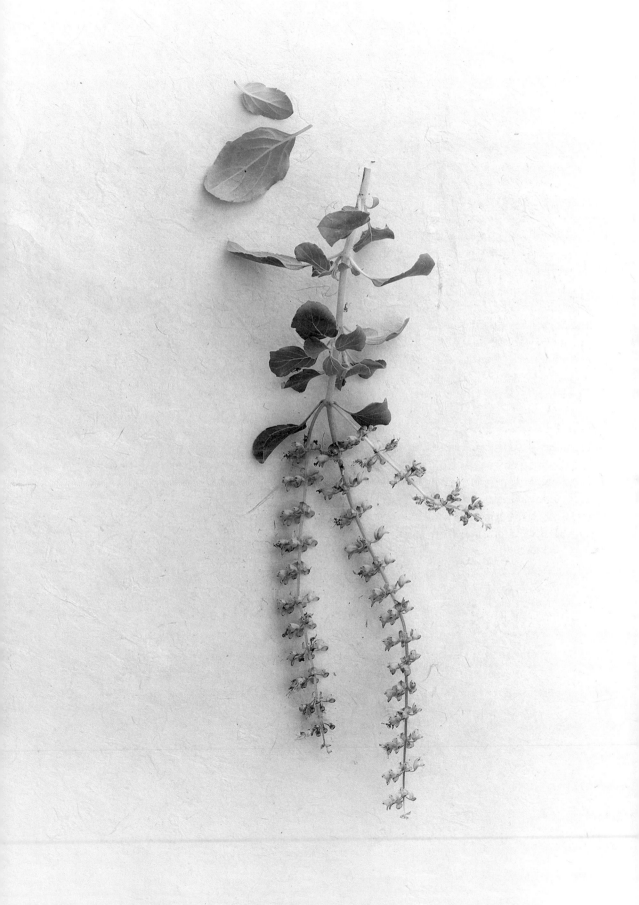

Hops

Humulus lupulus

Where Does It Grow?

Originally native to Europe and North America; today, hops are cultivated in many countries throughout the world.

What Does It Look Like?

A perennial climber with annual shoots (they grow anew each year), hops can stand up to 23 feet (7 m) tall. The shape of the leaves is reminiscent of grape leaves, but with a strongly serrated edge. The flowers of the female plants appear between July and August, and enlarge in the fall into attractive greenish yellow cones (hop cones).

Which Parts Are Used?

The hop cones.

What Does It Do?

Like valerian (see page 236), hops have exceptionally relaxing, sedative and soporific effects. Both are medicinal herbs and are often used in combination. Hop cones also contain estrogen-like substances and are therefore a favorite treatment for menopausal symptoms.

How Can I Use It?

Heart and Nerve Tonic (page 84). Hop pillows are also very popular; these are small cotton bags are filled with hop cones, which promote pleasant, restorative sleep.

What Do Scientists Think of It?

Numerous studies of the combination of hops and valerian confirm the positive effect of hops on sleep quality. The German Commission E and the European agency ESCOP (see page 155) also recommend hops for nervous restlessness, anxiety and sleep disorders. Unfortunately, trials of the effects on menopausal symptoms have not yet been held.

Caution

Unlike valerian, hops not only have a sedative effect, but are also soporific, meaning taking hops can affect your ability to react. You should therefore avoid products made with hops if you are planning to drive or operate machinery.

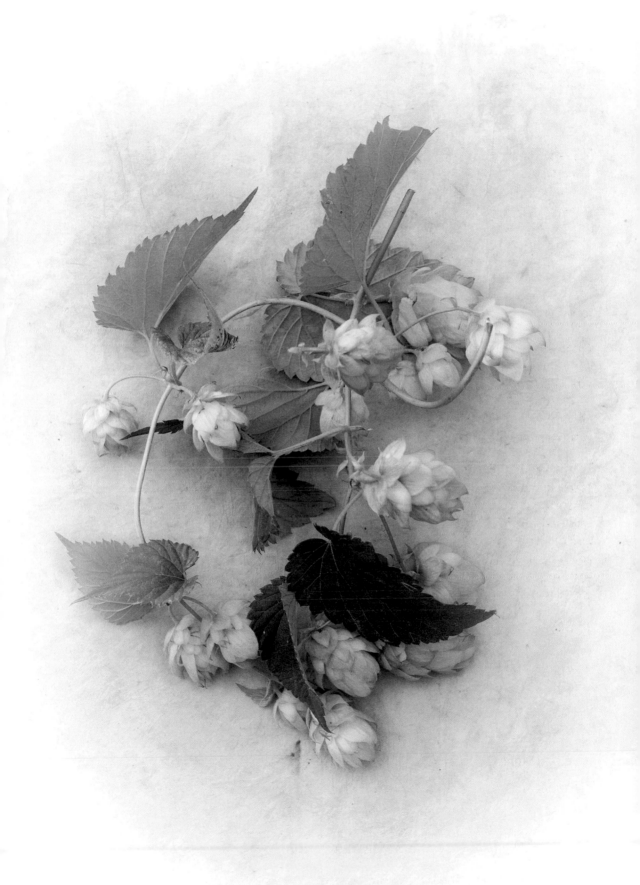

Horseradish

Armoracia rusticana

Where Does It Grow?
Originally from southeastern Europe; today, horseradish is cultivated around the world.

What Does It Look Like?
Horseradish is a frost-hardy, strong perennial plant, with large oval leaves that show prominent veins. From May to July, numerous strongly scented, small, white flowers open at the top of the stems, which can reach up to 4 feet (1.2 m) in height. The thick, woody, tapered root can grow to 20 inches (50 cm) long. It is harvested from fall into the following spring.

Which Parts Are Used?
The root (fresh or dried).

What Does It Do?
If you grate or cut horseradish, you'll instantly smell and feel the mustard oils it contains. The root owes not only its pungency but also its superb effect on the respiratory tract to these oils. Horseradish is also known for its digestion-boosting qualities, and because it stimulates blood flow, this unassuming root is often used externally in the form of ointments to treat gout and rheumatism.

How Can I Use It?
Horseradish Cough Linctus (page 66).

What Do Scientists Think of It?
The antibacterial action of horseradish has been proven in numerous studies, and this is why both the German Commission E and the European agency ESCOP (see page 155) recommend horseradish for colds and urinary tract infections. They also recommend external use of the root to treat mild muscle pains.

Caution
Because of its pungency, horseradish preparations are not suitable for small children or people who suffer from intestinal ulcers or kidney inflammation.

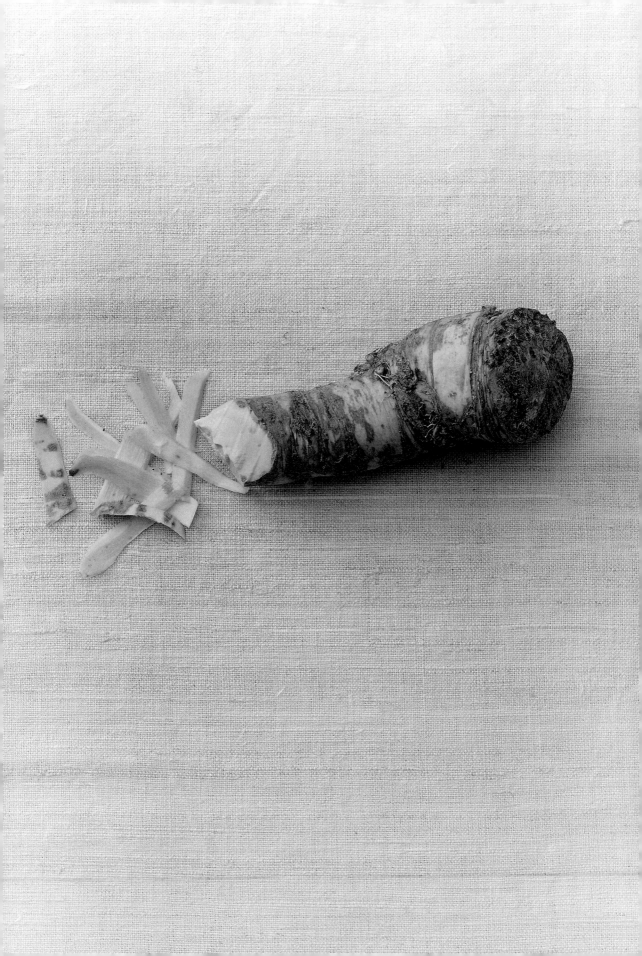

Lavender

Lavandula angustifolia

Where Does It Grow?
Originally from Mediterranean countries; today, lavender can be found in gardens all over the world.

What Does It Look Like?
A perennial subshrub (dwarf shrub) with upright, strongly scented stalks. The narrow, $1\frac{1}{2}$- to 2-inch (4 to 5 cm) long leaves, often with curled margins, are initially gray-blue, later green. The long-stemmed, violet flowers are in glorious bloom from June to August.

Which Parts Are Used?
The flowers.

What Does It Do?
Lavender has a relaxing effect on the muscles and the mind, thus helping fight stomach cramps, restlessness and difficulty falling asleep. Used externally, it helps treat rheumatism and wounds that are not healing well.

How Can I Use It?
Lavender Oil (page 96), Roll-On Lavender (page 102), Anti–Stretch Mark Oil (page 116), Breastfeeding Tea (page 119) and Tea Tree Oil Mouthwash (page 145).

What Do Scientists Think of It?
The German Commission E (see page 155) recommends lavender for anxiety, difficulty falling asleep, and nervous stomach and bowel complaints. In 2010, pharmacological trials at the University of Frankfurt, Germany, proved that a lavender preparation had the same effect on anxiety as conventional psychotherapeutic drugs.

Caution
In rare cases, lavender essential oil can cause an allergic reaction. There are no other restrictions on the herb's use.

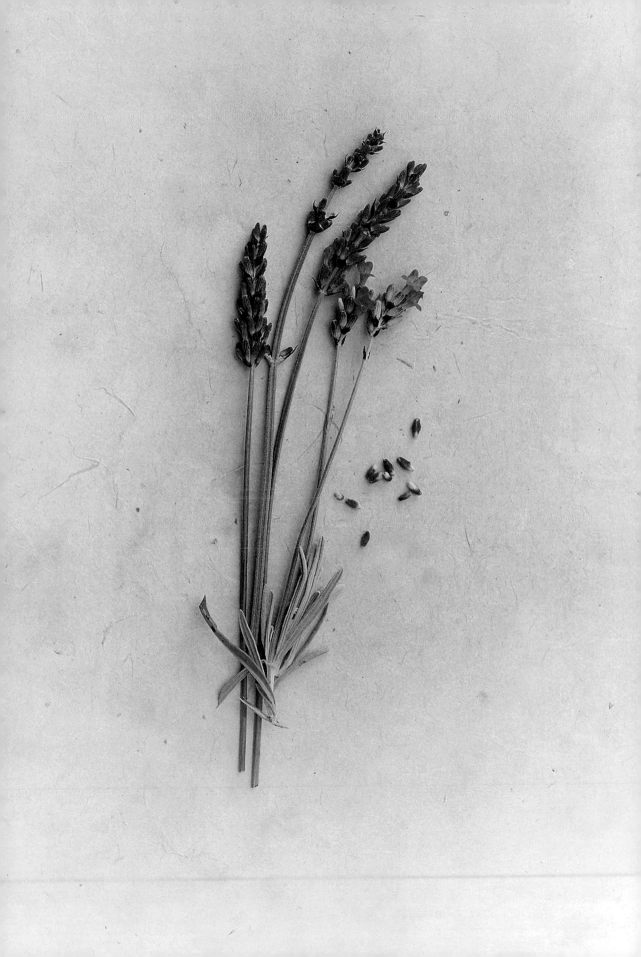

Lemon

Citrus medica or Citrus limonum

Where Does It Grow?
Around the world, in subtropical or tropical climatic zones.

What Does It Look Like?
Fast-growing, the lemon tree grows to be up to 16 feet (5 m) tall. The young shoots of this evergreen tree are covered in thorns. The elongated, oval, leathery and shiny green leaves are slightly serrated along the margins. The tree forms beautiful white and delicately scented flowers throughout the year. Within a year, the flowers develop into the well-known yellow fruits. Under its yellow, oily skin, each fruit has eight to 10 segments, separated by membranes, that contain the acidic flesh.

Which Parts Are Used?
The fruit's flesh and zest.

What Does It Do?
Thanks to its high vitamin C content, the lemon is the perfect household remedy for colds. In addition, it has antibacterial and detoxifying properties. Amazingly, despite its acidic flavor, lemon helps fight acid reflux, thanks to its alkaline components.

How Can I Use It?
Lemon Poultice (page 78), Garlic Drink (page 132) and Fig Syrup (page 142). I also swear by drinking 1 to 2 cups (250 to 500 mL) hot lemon water per day as a cold remedy. To make it, add the juice of one lemon to a generous ¾ cup (200 mL) hot (not boiling) water and sweeten with honey to taste.

What Do Scientists Think of It?
We've known for a long time that vitamin C is healthy. Several early studies have been able to demonstrate that the active substances in lemons have cancer cell–inhibiting powers, and more research is under way.

Caution
If you are allergic to lemons, you should obviously refrain from using any lemon-based preparations.

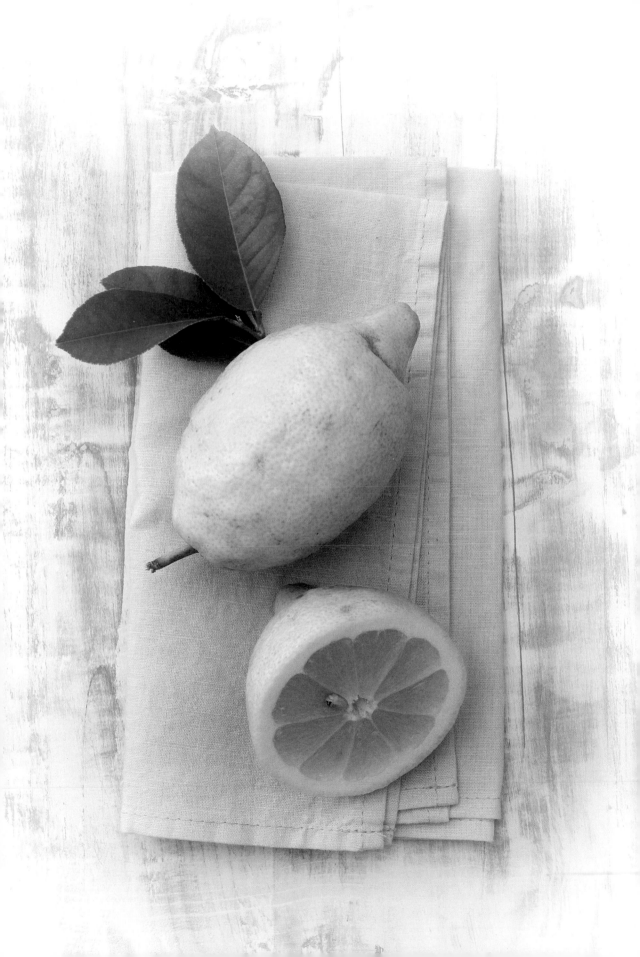

Lemon Balm (Melissa)

Melissa officinalis

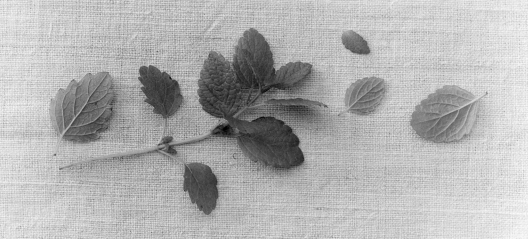

Where Does It Grow?

Originally a native of the Mediterranean region and western Asia; today, lemon balm is cultivated throughout Europe and in North America.

What Does It Look Like?

A perennial herb that grows up to 2¾ feet (90 cm) tall, with upright branching stems and light green, oval leaves that are irregularly toothed along the margins. The white to pinkish-red, small, lipped flowers open from July to August. The entire plant smells of lemon, hence its common name, lemon balm.

Which Parts Are Used?

The leaves.

What Does It Do?

Lemon balm is highly rated not only because it calms, balances mood and relieves anxiety, but also because it's used to treat menstrual and menopausal difficulties.

The herb boosts digestion, alleviates stomach cramps and is effective against colds. Used externally, it kills the virus that causes cold sores.

How Can I Use It?

Heart and Nerve Tonic (page 84), Lemon Balm Spirit (page 94), Breastfeeding Tea (page 119) and Anti–Cold Sore Balm (page 144). To make a simple tea, place 1 tsp (5 mL) fresh or dried lemon balm in a cup, pour a generous ¾ cup (200 mL) boiling water over top, then cover and let steep for 10 minutes.

What Do Scientists Think of It?

The German Commission E (see page 155) endorses lemon balm for anxiety-induced wakefulness, and for mild stomach and bowel complaints. ESCOP (see page 155) also recommends the herb for tension, anxiety and mental confusion. It also recommends external use of lemon balm to treat cold sores.

Linden Tree (Lime Tree or Basswood Tree)

Tilia spp.

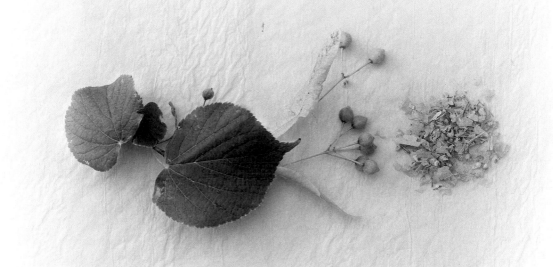

Where Does It Grow?
Europe.

What Does It Look Like?
This deciduous tree grows up to 130 feet (40 m) tall (depending on the variety), with large, heart-shaped leaves with serrated edges. Yellowish, scented panicles of flowers open in June. They are fused with a conspicuous elongated bract that later serves as a flying aid for the pea-size fruits.

Which Parts Are Used?
The dried flowers; for medicinal purposes, the flowers of the large-leaved linden are used most often.

What Does It Do?
Linden flowers increase the body's defenses, promote perspiration and lower fevers. In addition, they have a calming effect during stressful experiences and reduce hypertension caused by nervous disorders.

How Can I Use It?
Anti-Flu Tea (page 74) and Sinus Tea (page 77). You can also make a simple tea from linden flowers: place 1 tsp (5 mL) flowers in a cup, pour a generous ¾ cup (200 mL) boiling water over top, then cover and let steep for 10 minutes. If you have a cold, start drinking the tea as soon as the first symptoms appear; it will boost your immune system.

What Do Scientists Think of It?
The German Commission E (see page 155) recommends linden flowers to treat colds and dry chest coughs.

Caution
There is no scientific evidence on the use of linden during pregnancy or breastfeeding, so consult your physician before using it.

Marigold (Calendula)

Calendula officinalis

Where Does It Grow?

Originally from Eastern Europe; today, cultivated across the globe.

What Does It Look Like?

An annual, with 12- to 20-inch (30 to 50 cm) tall, upright stems covered in short hairs. The light to medium green, oval leaves are also covered in downy hairs. From June to October, the plant forms long-lasting bright yellow to orange flower heads.

Which Parts Are Used?

The flowers and the leaves.

What Does It Do?

Marigold essential oil has anti-inflammatory properties and suppresses the growth of bacteria and fungi. Its active substances speed up healing processes in the skin and help heal wounds to the mucous membranes. It also prevents inflammation, which is why the flower has long been a mainstay of the natural pharmacy. Marigold is only rarely used internally today, although it does have a regularizing effect on menstruation.

How Can I Use It?

Wound Cleanser (page 57) and Sea Salt Nasal Spray (page 70).

What Do Scientists Think of It?

Both the German Commission E and the European agency ESCOP (see page 155) endorse the external use of marigold for inflammations of the mucous membranes and skin, as well as an aid for wound healing.

Caution

If you are allergic to daisy-like flowers, you shouldn't use marigold preparations. Other than that, no negative side effects of the herb are known.

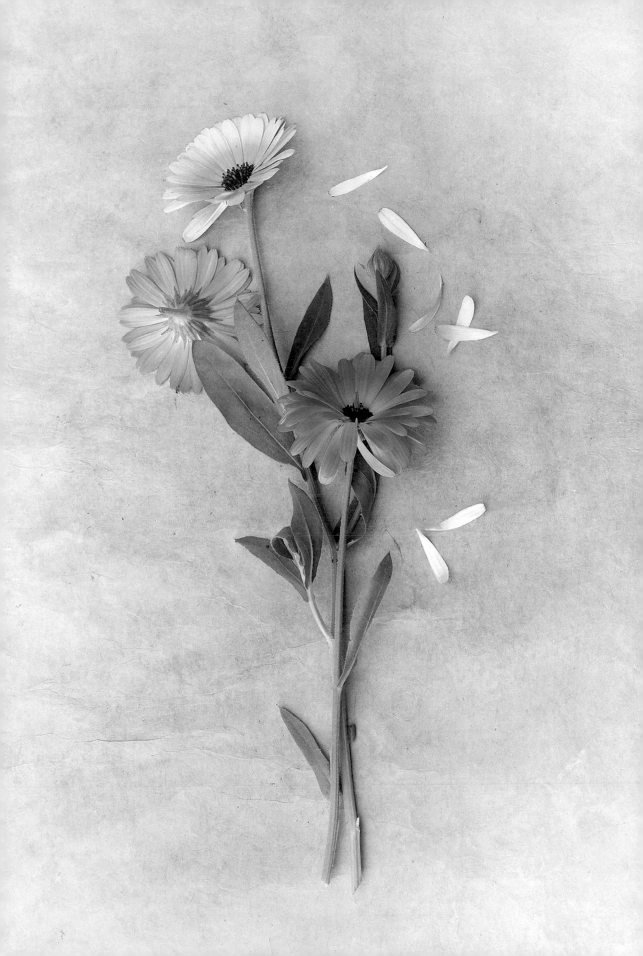

Marjoram
Origanum majorana

....

Where Does It Grow?
Native to Asia, but grown since antiquity across the Mediterranean region.

What Does It Look Like?
This perennial (in gardens usually annual or biennial) plant belongs to the mint family. The oval leaves are covered in short downy hairs and grow in opposed pairs, on tall, thin stems up to 20 inches (50 cm) in height. The small white to reddish flowers open from June to September in ball-shaped spikes. Botanically, marjoram is a close relative of oregano, thyme and sage.

Which Parts Are Used?
The whole plant.

What Does It Do?
Marjoram clears air passages and alleviates cold symptoms. It also has a calming and balancing effect on the nervous system. In the digestive system, marjoram acts as an antispasmodic and stimulates digestion; it also prevents flatulence and colic. For this reason, and because of its strong aroma, it is included in many spice mixtures for cured meats, such as salami or liverwurst. If used as an additive in a steam bath, marjoram can relieve the symptoms of a cold; it also helps remove skin impurities.

How Can I Use It?
Marjoram Ointment (page 37) and Sinus Tea (page 77). A tea made from fresh or dried marjoram works as an alcohol-free digestive drink after a rich meal. Place 1 tsp (5 mL) marjoram leaves in a cup, pour a generous ¾ cup (200 mL) boiling water over top, then cover and let steep for 10 minutes.

What Do Scientists Think of It?
Unfortunately, the traditional lore about this plant's healing powers has not yet been substantiated by scientific trials.

Caution
Like all other medicinal herbal teas, marjoram tea should not be drunk for more than six weeks in a row. Otherwise it may lead to headaches. This tea is not suitable for pregnant women.

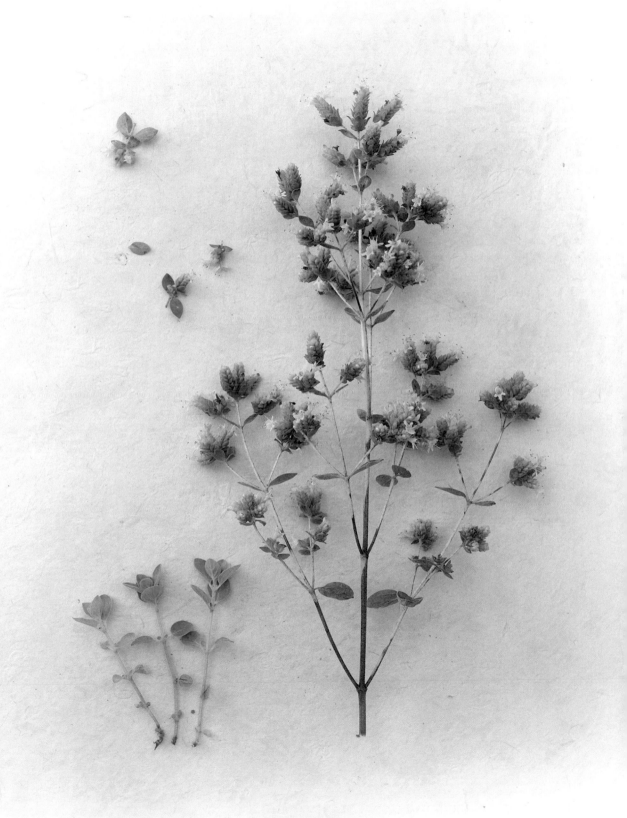

Meadowsweet

Filipendula ulmaria

Where Does It Grow?

Europe.

What Does It Look Like?

This herbaceous perennial grows to 6½ feet (2 m) tall. Bright green, feathered leaves with clearly visible veins and white on the undersides grow from the reddish stems. The white flower clusters appear from June or July to August. They exude an intensely sweet scent, especially in the evening.

Which Parts Are Used?

The flowers, leaves and roots.

What Does It Do?

Meadowsweet contains salicylic acid, the active ingredient in Aspirin (also called acetylsalicylic acid, or ASA, generically). Just like its chemical counterpart, this herb alleviates pain. However, unlike Aspirin, meadowsweet protects the stomach lining and reduces the production of stomach acids. (Often, nature is cleverer than humans.) In addition, the herb also has anti-inflammatory, fever-reducing, antirheumatic and diuretic properties.

How Can I Use It?

Anti-Flu Tea (page 74) and Sinus Tea (page 77). If you're suffering from gastritis or acid reflux, you can drink meadowsweet tea for its antacid and anti-inflammatory action. To make a simple tea, place 1 tsp (5 mL) meadowsweet in a cup, pour a generous ¾ cup (200 mL) boiling water over top, then cover and let steep for 10 minutes. For rheumatic joint complaints, moisten a cloth in meadowsweet tea and place the compress on the affected joint for 30 minutes.

What Do Scientists Think of It?

The German Commission E (see page 155) endorses meadowsweet as a complement to conventional therapies for treating colds.

Caution

If you are allergic to salicylic acid, avoid meadowsweet. There is no evidence, as yet, about the effects of using meadowsweet during pregnancy and breastfeeding, so you are advised to not use the herb during these times.

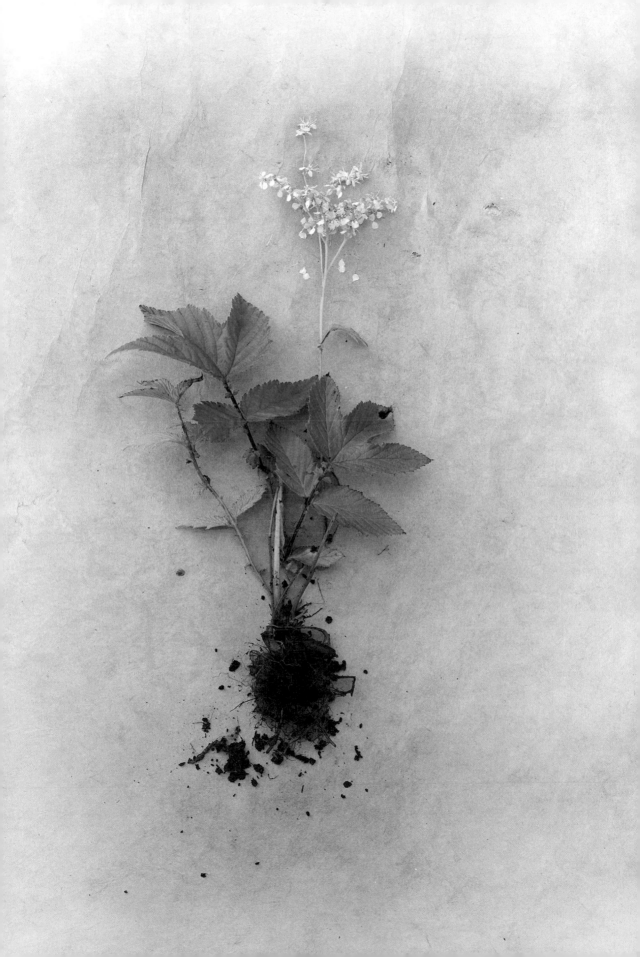

Moringa
Moringa oleifera

Where Does It Grow?
Originally from the Himalayan region of northern India, the plant has since spread to many tropical and subtropical areas.

What Does It Look Like?
Moringa is a fast-growing tree from the Moringaceae family (ben nut trees). Its pale green leaves are feathery, with two or three lobes. The flowers are white to cream-colored and smell faintly of violets. They develop into long fruit capsules after fertilization. The capsules burst when ripe and release the seeds.

Which Parts Are Used?
Leaves, fruits, seeds and roots; the roots contain the active substances in such high concentrations that their use should be restricted to physicians and natural health practitioners.

What Does It Do?
Thanks to its high content of vitamins, minerals, trace elements and essential amino acids, moringa is an ideal food for anyone with above-average nutrient requirements, such as breastfeeding or menopausal women, the elderly or people experiencing chronic stress or chronic illness. In Africa and Asia, the plant is used to counter nutritional deficiencies in children and the elderly. Moringa is extremely rich in protein, so it is also perfectly suited to vegetarians.

Besides its nutritional benefits, moringa has an antioxidant effect that is higher than that of any other plant. It is therefore capable of disarming considerably more free radicals; this effectively protects cells and cell tissue from damage and strengthens the body's defenses against infection. Thanks to their antibiotic and anti-inflammatory properties, moringa roots are traditionally used to treat gout and rheumatism.

How Can I Use It?
Moringa Smoothie (page 149). You can also eat the raw leaves in salads, cook the leaves in soups or take dried powdered leaves as a nutritional supplement. The beanlike fruits can be eaten raw or cooked as a vegetable; they are very nutritious and have an asparagus-like flavor. The seeds can be cooked like peas; usually, they are roasted and pressed to make moringa oil.

What Do Scientists Think of It?
There have been more than 700 studies on the beneficial effects of moringa. In the United States especially, the plant is now rated as a high-grade nutritional supplement.

Caution
Although moringa is traditionally taken during pregnancy in India and Africa, no studies have been carried out on the potential side effects. Pregnant women are therefore advised to avoid it.

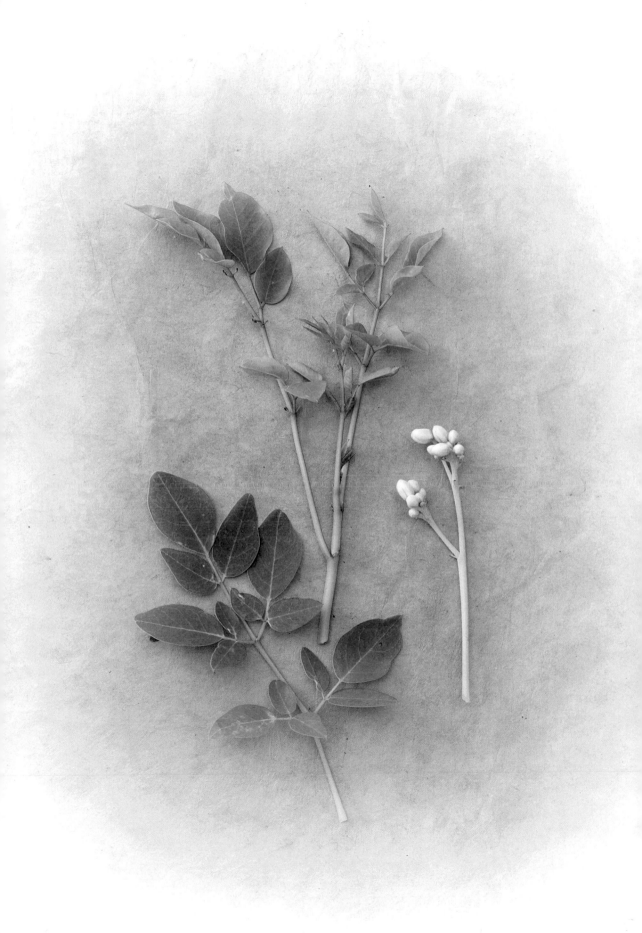

Neem Tree

Azadirachta indica

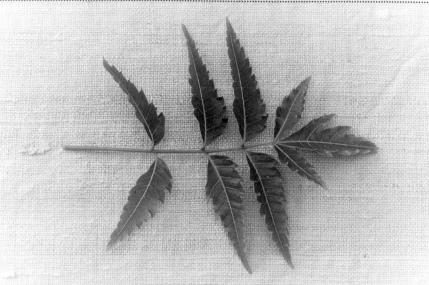

Where Does It Grow?

Originally native to southwest India and Burma; today, neem trees grow in many tropical and subtropical countries.

What Does It Look Like?

The neem tree is an evergreen tree with a large crown and elongated, feathery leaves that can reach up to 16 inches (40 cm) in length. The small white flowers grow in panicles, with a scent reminiscent of jasmine. After flowering, the tree forms olive-like neem fruits, from which neem oil is pressed.

Which Parts Are Used?

The fruits, which are pressed to make oil.

What Does It Do?

Neem oil is used for pest control, and as an insecticide to fight mites on plants. It is also helpful for fighting pests that plague dogs and cats (such as fleas), as well as for treating head lice in humans.

How Can I Use It?

Anti-Lice Shampoo (page 43).

What Do Scientists Think of It?

Studies have scientifically demonstrated that neem oil fights parasites such as head lice. It was initially presumed to fight household dust mites, but its efficacy has not been confirmed. In animal trials, neem oil shows beneficial action against malaria; this is currently being investigated further.

Caution

No side effects are known for external application of neem oil. However, it has a strong, earthy, nut-like smell that is not to everyone's liking. There are no relevant studies on internal use, so you're advised to refrain from ingesting neem oil.

Parsley
Petroselinum crispum

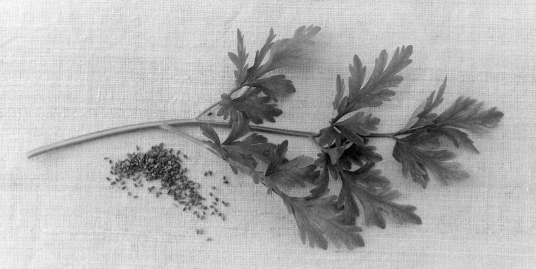

Where Does It Grow?
Native to the Mediterranean; today, parsley is cultivated in many places around the world.

What Does It Look Like?
A biennial plant, parsley has dark green, flat or curly leaves, depending on the variety. In the plant's second year, flowers appear between June and July, followed in fall by small, brown, egg-shaped seeds.

Which Parts Are Used?
The leaves and seeds.

What Does It Do?
Parsley acts as a diuretic and therefore has been used in folk medicine for minor bladder complaints. It assists digestion, induces menstruation and inhibits inflammation. Increasingly, it is also being used to treat menopausal complaints. Chew a few stems for a quick bad breath remedy (especially to help fight garlic breath). Rub a few leaves on the skin to alleviate itching from mosquito bites.

How Can I Use It?
Parsley Poultice (page 36).

What Do Scientists Think of It?
In 2012, scientists at the University of Missouri in the United States were able to prove in animal tests that a component of parsley essential oil inhibits breast cancer tumor cells. A Japanese study ascribes phytohormonal properties to parsley that are similar to those of the soybean.

Caution
Pregnant women should use caution when consuming parsley; ingested in large quantities, it may cause the onset of labor. People with acute kidney infections should never consume parsley.

Pomegranate

Punica granatum

Where Does It Grow?

Native to Iran; today, pomegranates are also cultivated in northern India, western and central Asia, the Mediterranean region and North America.

What Does It Look Like?

The pomegranate tree is a small deciduous tree, with showy orange-red to light yellow bell-shaped flowers that ripen into hard, dark orange to red fruits that are about the size of apples. Inside the fruit, several hundred angular arils lie in chambers; each aril is filled with a transparent pink to red, juicy pulp, which surrounds a large seed.

Which Parts Are Used?

The fleshy seed coverings (arils).

What Does It Do?

The pomegranate's active compounds—flavonoids, potassium, calcium, vitamin C, iron and polyphenols—are able to capture free radicals and can thus prevent calcification and the formation of harmful deposits on blood vessel walls. This means they protect us from degenerative age-related diseases, such as cardiovascular disease, high blood pressure, dementia and cancer.

How Can I Use It?

Pomegranate Juice (page 137) and Moringa Smoothie (page 149). You can also simply eat the arils; try them in a fruit salad or as a dessert garnish.

What Do Scientists Think of It?

Some 250 scientific studies have been conducted around the world on the health benefits of pomegranates. Many positive effects have been demonstrated. Among them are that pomegranate juice significantly slows down the rise in prostate-specific antigen (PSA) levels in prostate cancer. (PSA is the most important tumor and progress marker for this type of cancer.) Pomegranate juice can also improve the blood's antioxidant protection by more than 100%. It also can reduce the formation of beta-amyloid protein in the brain by half; this protein plays a decisive part in the development of Alzheimer's disease. As well, pomegranate juice can prevent or delay the onset of arthritis, or substantially reduce the severity of the disease. Finally, the juice also reduces the amounts of harmful deposits in the carotid artery and increases blood flow within the heart muscle, therefore reducing the number of angina pectoris attacks.

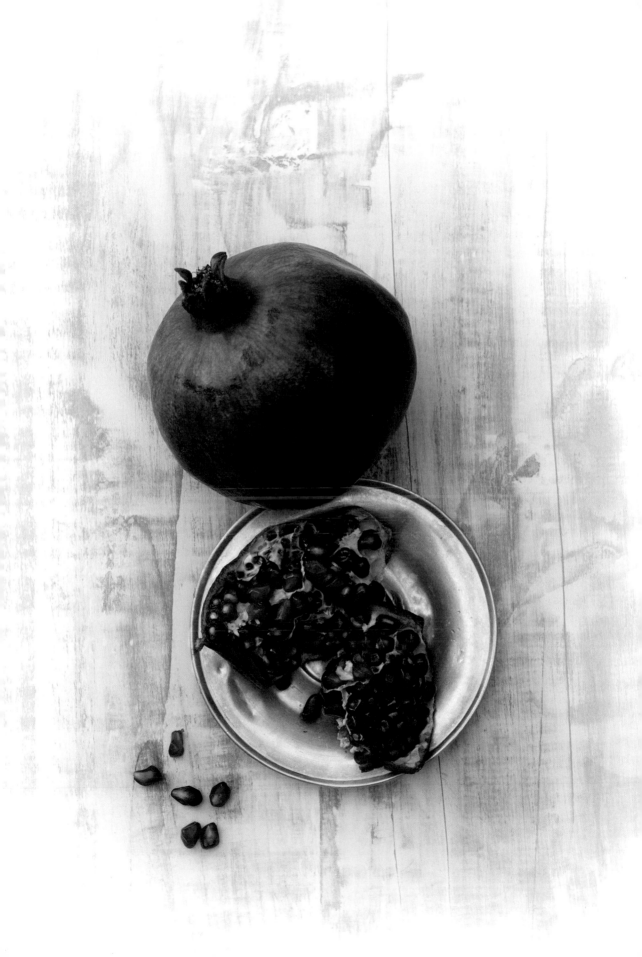

Potato

Solanum tuberosum

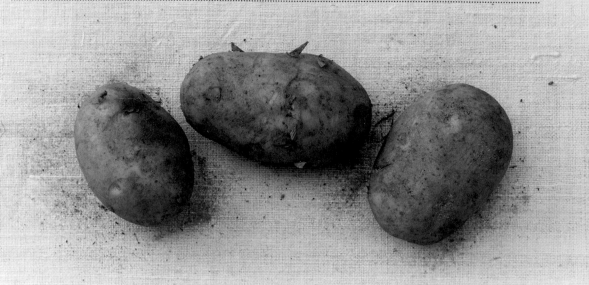

Where Does It Grow?

A native of the Andes region of South America; today, potatoes are grown virtually everywhere in world.

What Does It Look Like?

A member of the Solanaceae family, the potato plant has large, feathered leaves. Small, bell-shaped white, pink or violet flowers form at the end of July. The underground offshoots thicken in early summer and grow into tubers, or what we call potatoes.

Which Parts Are Used?

The tubers.

What Does It Do?

Potatoes are much more than just an inexpensive way to satisfy your hunger. Thanks to their alkaline-rich components, they fight acidification in the body (especially the stomach). They are rich in healthy fibers that calm the stomach and bowels. Used externally, they draw inflammations out of the skin and boost blood flow.

How Can I Use It?

Potato Decoction (page 114).

What Do Scientists Think of It?

In 2011, Dr. Joe Vinson, a professor at the University of Scranton in Pennsylvania, examined the effect of the potato on the health of 18 overweight study participants who suffered from high blood pressure. The participants ate six to eight small, unpeeled potatoes twice a day for one month. As a result, their blood pressure fell by up to 4.3%.

Caution

Avoid all green parts of the potato plant; they are toxic, because they contain the alkaloid solanine.

Psyllium (Fleawort)

Plantago ovata or *Plantago afra*

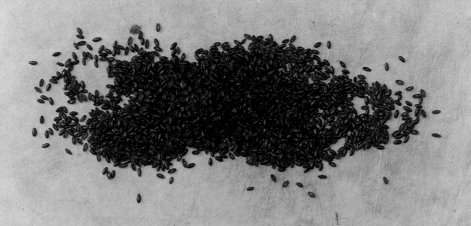

Where Does It Grow?

Originally native to Mediterranean countries and western Asia; today the plant also grows in Israel, Spain, Brazil, Russia and Japan.

What Does It Look Like?

Psyllium is an herbaceous annual plant, up to 20 inches (50 cm) tall, with a ground-hugging rosette of elongated leaves. Its white flower spikes appear from April to July.

Which Parts Are Used?

The seeds.

What Does It Do?

The seeds help treat constipation in two ways: the fibre in the seed husks "bulks up" the stool, and the mucins contained in the seeds ensure a soft consistency. In the case of diarrhea, however, psyllium seeds have the opposite effect, bringing about firmer stools.

How Can I Use It?

Fig Syrup (page 142). You can also take psyllium seeds on their own, with plenty of water (see page 148).

What Do Scientists Think of It?

A number of studies have been conducted; among them, some have demonstrated that anyone who takes 0.35 oz (10 g) of psyllium seeds daily over a period of two weeks can significantly increase bowel activity. In the 1990s, it was also proven that psyllium seeds could lower cholesterol levels.

Caution

Psyllium seeds should not be taken at the same time as other medications, because the mucins in psyllium can impair their effect. A gap of one hour between taking psyllium and other medications is ideal. The recommended daily dose of 0.35 to 1.4 oz (10 to 40 g) should not be exceeded. In the case of intestinal obstruction, or pathological narrowing or inflammation in the gastrointestinal tract, psyllium seeds should not be taken at all.

Pu'erh Tea (Pu'er Tea)

Camellia sinensis

Where Does It Grow?

Originated in the area around Pu'er City in the Chinese province of Yunnan.

What Does It Look Like?

A compact, heavily branched, large shrub or small tree with leathery, shiny, dark green leaves, partly covered in hairs on the undersides. Depending on location, white flowers with yellow stamens appear in late winter, summer or fall.

Which Parts Are Used?

The leaves.

What Does It Do?

Pu'erh tea has been used as a digestive aid since ancient times; drinking it after a rich meal is still a must in China. Traditional Chinese medicine also values pu'erh as a remedy after alcohol consumption because it detoxifies the liver. It is also said to help lower blood cholesterol levels.

How Can I Use It?

Hangover Tea (page 98).

What Do Scientists Think of It?

Scientific evidence does not exist for every benefit this tea is said to offer. This is the case, for example, with the assertion that pu'erh boosts fat burning. The tea's cholesterol-lowering action has so far only been demonstrated in animal experiments. However, it is considered confirmed that the secondary plant compounds found in high amounts in this tea protect the body from free radicals, stimulate the immune system and inhibit inflammation.

Caution

Pu'erh tea does not contain as much caffeine as coffee, but you should still consume it in moderation. Drink a maximum of three cups per day.

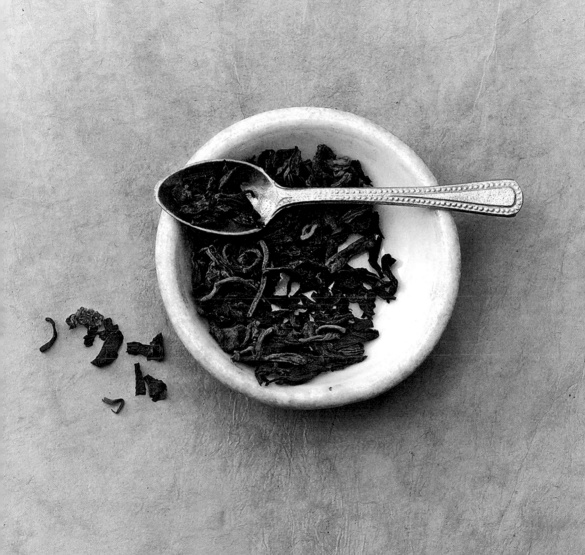

Rose

Rosa spp.

Where Does It Grow?
Around the world.

What Does It Look Like?
There are hundreds of different types of roses that differ in growth habits, types of flowers and colors. The stems and branches are covered in thorns. The usually oval feathery leaves have five leaflets with serrated margins that are green in most species but red in others. The flowers grow in clusters (or, in some species, as individual flowers) from the sides and/or ends of the branches. Depending on species and variety, roses flower from June through late fall. The flowers ripen into decorative fruits called rose hips.

Which Parts Are Used?
The flowers (of scented roses only).

What Does It Do?
In the Middle Ages, rose tea was taken for headaches, uterine pain and diarrhea because of its contracting and cooling properties. In modern times, roses are used mainly in external applications to treat insect stings, skin diseases, and swollen or inflamed eyes. Rose oil is also a popular ingredient in skin care preparations; for example, to treat pregnancy-induced stretch marks. The queen of flowers plays an important role in aromatherapy as well: inhaling rose scent is said to help relieve tension and restore peace of mind.

How Can I Use It?
Rose Gel (page 38), Rose Powder (page 86) and Perineal Massage Oil (page 118).

What Do Scientists Think of It?
As part of a study, gynecologists at the University of Paris, France, discovered that the regular inhalation of rose scent positively affected a woman's hormonal balance and alleviated menstrual and menopausal complaints. In another study, scientists at the University of Lübeck, Germany, asked participants to learn new content while inhaling rose scent, then sent them to bed. Some of the test participants slept in scent-free rooms, the others in rose-scented rooms. The result was that 97% of the study's rose-scent group recalled what they had learned earlier; of the non-rose-scent group, only 85% remembered the new information.

Caution
There are no known side effects for the use of rose preparations, but you should always look for high-quality products. For herbal treatments and recipes, use only unsprayed rose petals and natural organic rose essential oil (though this essential oil is very expensive at $200 to $700 per 1 oz/30 mL in North America). Synthetic rose scent is much cheaper but has no healing powers whatsoever.

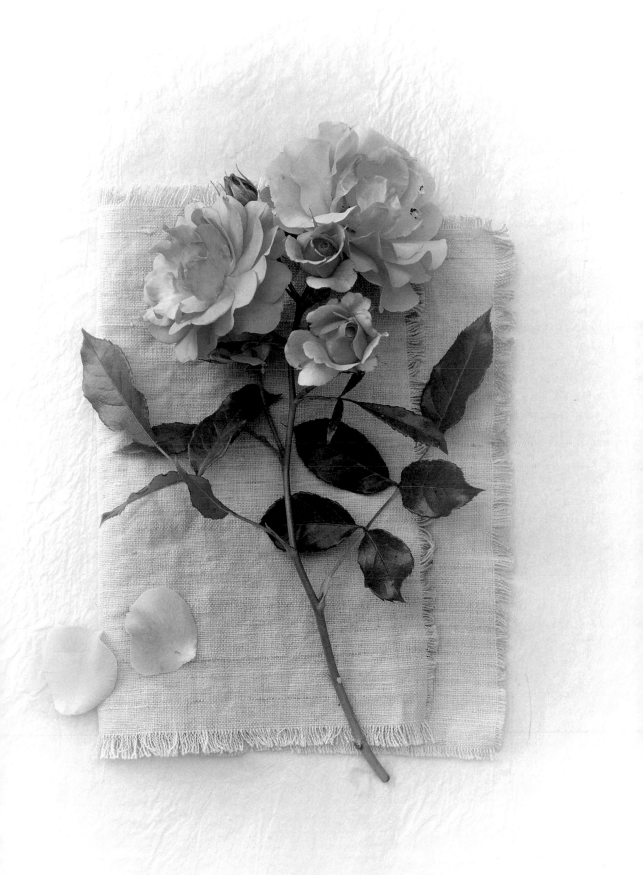

Rosemary

Rosmarinus officinalis

Where Does It Grow?

Originally from the Mediterranean region; today, cultivated throughout Europe and many other parts of the world.

What Does It Look Like?

A perennial evergreen shrub, heavily branched, rosemary grows up to 5 feet (1.5 m) tall. The up to 1½-inch (4 cm) long, narrow, leathery leaves are dark green on top, and silvery white and downy below. They roll toward the underside and, at first glance, look like pine needles. Many small, light blue flowers open between March and May, and sometimes a second time in September.

Which Parts Are Used?

The leaves and flowers.

What Does It Do?

Taken internally, rosemary relaxes the digestive tract, which is why it is often used to treat spasms. It also strengthens the heart and boosts low blood pressure. Its scent improves concentration and the powers of recall. As a bath additive, it stimulates blood flow, alleviates rheumatic complaints, relaxes the muscles and animates the mind.

How Can I Use It?

Pine Rubbing Lotion (page 60), Hi There! Wake Up! Oil (page 99), Skin Toning Oil (page 107) and Rosemary Wine (page 134). For a rosemary bath, stir 10 drops of rosemary essential oil into a small carton of cream and add the mixture to hot bathwater. Relax in the water for 15 to 20 minutes.

What Do Scientists Think of It?

The German Commission E (see page 155) endorses the consumption of rosemary for digestive troubles and also recommends external use of the herb to supplement conventional therapies for circulatory disorders and rheumatic complaints.

Caution

Rosemary should not be consumed in large quantities during pregnancy or breastfeeding, because it may lead to uterine bleeding. Also refrain from taking a rosemary bath just before going to bed, because it will revive you (all other dosage formats are fine in the evening). Allergic reactions may occur, as with all plants from the Lamiaceae, or mint, family.

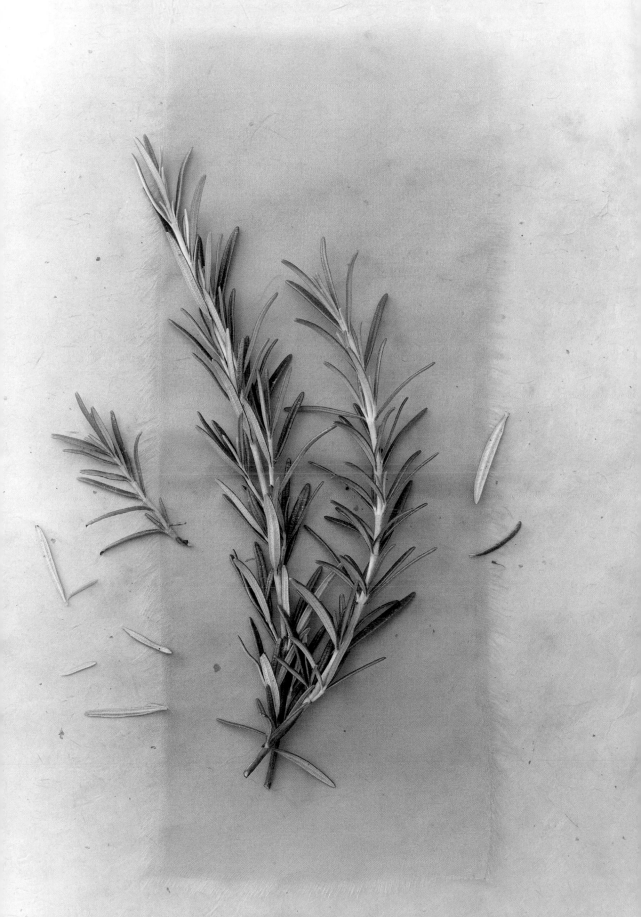

Sage
Salvia officinalis

Where Does It Grow?
Originally a native of the Mediterranean region, today, sage is grown in all temperate climatic regions.

What Does It Look Like?
Rosemary is a perennial evergreen branched subshrub of the Lamiaceae (mint) family, with woody stems whose upper parts are hairy. The felt-textured oval leaves are initially gray-green, later more silvery. Blue-violet, lipped flowers appear in the leaf axils from late spring.

Which Parts Are Used?
The leaves.

What Does It Do?
Thanks to its expectorant and antibacterial qualities, sage is highly rated in herbal medicine for the treatment of coughs, colds and sore throats. It has also proven successful for treating gastrointestinal complaints, diarrhea and lack of appetite. It is also used as a rinse or gargle for dental inflammations and injuries to the oral mucous membranes. Women have long relied on the herb to treat excessive perspiration, hot flashes and other menopausal complaints. Sage is also said to improve memory capacity.

How Can I Use It?
Sage Candy (page 58), Gargling Solution (page 72) and Rose Powder (page 86).

What Do Scientists Think of It?
Many smaller studies have confirmed that sage has antibacterial properties and inhibits sweat production. Both the German Commission E and the European agency ESCOP (see page 155) endorse taking sage for malfunctions of the gastrointestinal tract and for excessive perspiration. They endorse external use of sage for inflammations of the mouth and throat. Scientists are currently exploring the effect of sage on dementia.

Caution
Breastfeeding women should avoid sage because it inhibits lactation. Sage also contains small quantities of camphor and thujone, which can lead to cramps and dizziness if taken in excess. This risk, however, only applies to concentrated products (such as capsules or other pills). In tea and other watery applications, you don't have to worry about overdosing.

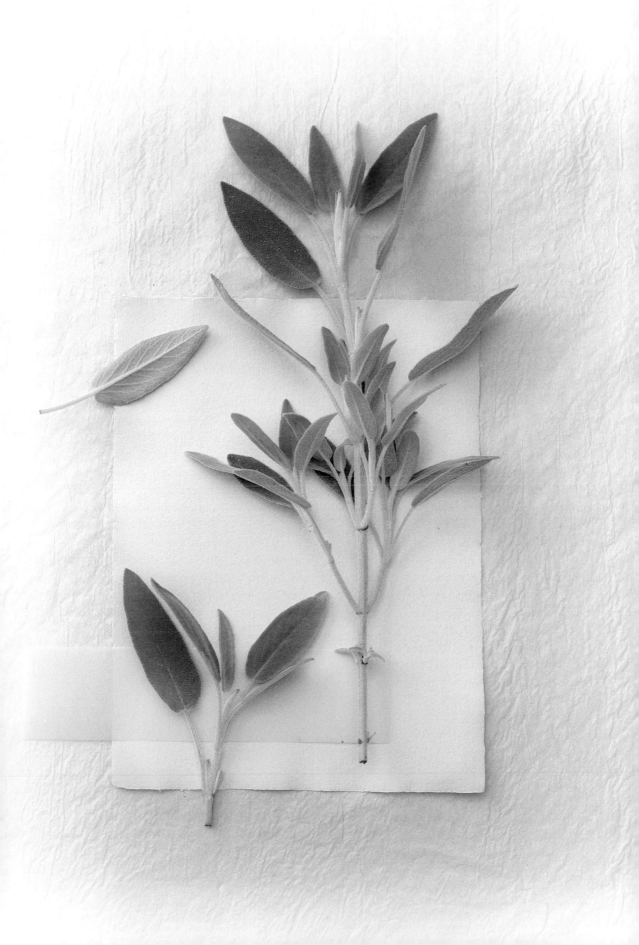

St. John's Wort

Hypericum perforatum

Where Does It Grow?
Europe and western Asia.

What Does It Look Like?
A perennial herb, St. John's wort grows up to 3 feet (1 m) tall. The reddish stems branch toward the top and produce small oval leaflets covered in oil glands. The golden yellow flowers appear from about mid-May and continue flowering into August.

Which Parts Are Used?
The whole flowering herb, especially the flowers.

What Does It Do?
Over many centuries, St. John's wort was used mainly for its wound-healing power. The red oil from the flower buds is considered an antiseptic and was used to treat both slow-healing wounds and burns (including sunburns). It was not until the 19th century that the herb's positive effect on mental health was discovered. St. John's wort contains hypericin and hyperforin, two substances that are beneficial for treating depression, anxiety and insomnia.

How Can I Use It?
St. John's Wort Oil (page 52), Heart and Nerve Tonic (page 84), St. John's Wort Tincture (page 92) and Perineal Massage Oil (page 118).

What Do Scientists Think of It?
In more than 30 studies, 5,000-plus participants suffering from light to moderate depression were treated with a high dose of St. John's wort extract. The results demonstrated that using St. John's wort as a remedy for depression is in no way inferior to using synthetic antidepressants. Unlike these, however, St. John's wort has no side effects.

Both the German Commission E and the European agency ESCOP (see page 155) endorse the use of St. John's wort for mild to moderate depression. Commission E also endorses external use of St. John's wort for burns and injuries.

Caution
St. John's wort can increase light sensitivity of the skin, even when used internally. If you are taking blood-thinning medication to stop clotting, consult your physician before ingesting this medicinal plant. There is no scientific evidence about use of St. John's wort during pregnancy or breastfeeding; if you are suffering from depression during these times, talk with your physician before taking it.

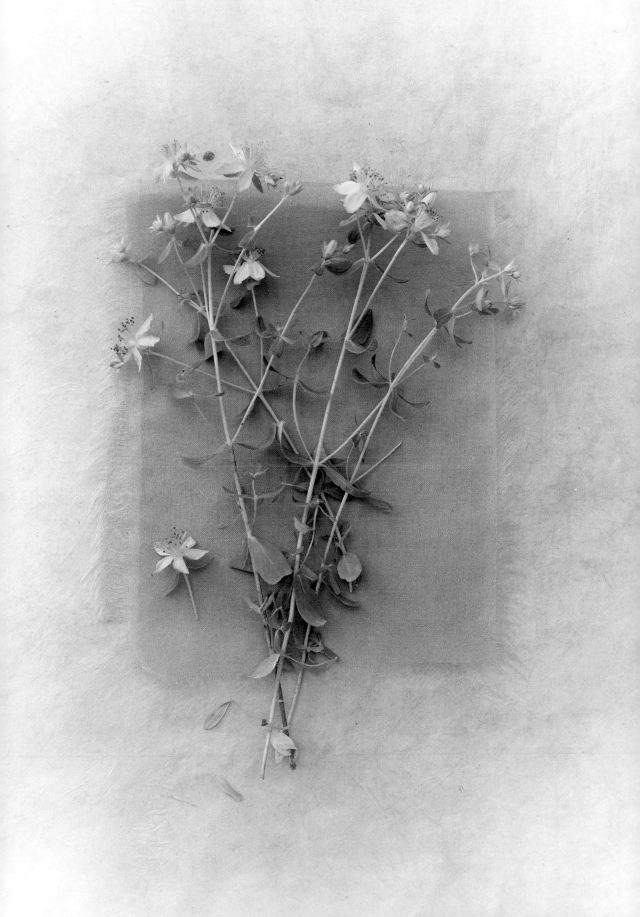

Silver Birch

Betula pendula

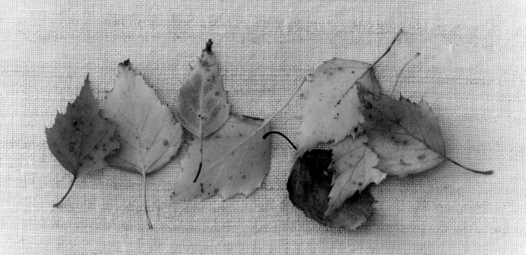

Where Does It Grow?
Europe and moderate climatic zones of Asia.

What Does It Look Like?
A deciduous tree that grows up to 100 feet (30 m) tall, the silver birch has white bark that peels off or turns black and hard. The dark green leaves are clearly lighter on the undersides; they have serrated margins.

Which Parts Are Used?
The dried leaves.

What Does It Do?
Silver birch leaves have dehydrating and diuretic properties, as well as a disinfectant effect, and are therefore used to treat inflammatory bladder and kidney diseases. They contain substances that help flush harmful substances out of the body, so they are also popular for treating gout and joint complaints, and as a component in detoxing teas. Silver birch leaves are also used externally to fight dandruff and alopecia.

How Can I Use It?
Spring Tea (page 95).

What Do Scientists Think of It?
In a large-scale study of people who suffered from cystitis and urethritis, 92% of participants rated the effect of silver birch leaf extract on their condition as good or very good. The German Commission E and the European agency ESCOP (see page 155) also endorse the use of silver birch for kidney stones and diseases of the urinary tract, and as a supplementary treatment for rheumatic complaints.

Caution
Silver birch leaves must not be used by people who are experiencing fluid retention due to impaired kidney or heart function. The same applies to pregnant and breastfeeding women; we are still waiting for scientific evaluation of the use of silver birch in these situations.

Speedwell

Veronica officinalis

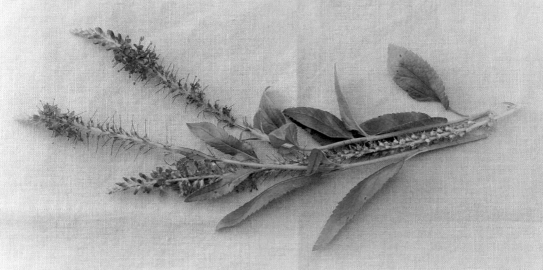

Where Does It Grow?
Europe, North America and northern Asia.

What Does It Look Like?
Speedwell is an herbaceous perennial that grows up to 12 inches (30 cm) tall, with grayish-green, slightly hairy stems and toothed leaves. The bright, light blue or pale violet flowers generally appear from late spring into summer.

Which Parts Are Used?
The whole flowering herb.

What Does It Do?
Speedwell was very popular in the Middle Ages and was used in a variety of cases; it was even thought to protect against the plague by physicians at that time. Speedwell stimulates digestion and the metabolism, promotes expectoration of phlegm during coughing spells and cleanses the blood. It is also indispensable for skin diseases because it alleviates itching. The plant is often combined with other herbs because it tastes slightly bitter.

How Can I Use It?
Spring Tea (page 95) and Virility Tea (page 126).

What Do Scientists Think of It?
No scientific studies have been carried out on the use of speedwell yet.

Spruce

Picea spp.

Where Does It Grow?
Throughout Europe and other northern temperate and boreal regions of the world.

What Does It Look Like?
An evergreen tree, with a scaly, brownish-red trunk, spruce trees may grow up to 200 feet (60 m) tall, with a diameter of up to 6 ½ feet (2 m). The branches form a conical crown. The angular, pointed needles are connected to the branches via short stems and arranged in a spiral shape. The light green buds (shoots) are egg- to ball-shaped.

Which Parts Are Used?
Young shoots, needles and resin.

What Does It Do?
The tender young shoots of the spruce are used to treat diseases of the respiratory tract and for rheumatic pain. Spruce essential oil stimulates circulation.

How Can I Use It?
Pine Rubbing Lotion (page 60), Spruce Bath Salts (page 62) and Rheumatism Tincture (page 136). Spruce essential oil is an expectorant, so it is excellent if used in a steam bath (add three or four drops to the hot water).

What Do Scientists Think of It?
The German Commission E (see page 155) recommends spruce for respiratory diseases, rheumatic complaints and neuralgic pain.

Caution
Don't use spruce in a bath if your skin is damaged. Stop using spruce if you are diagnosed with whooping cough or asthma.

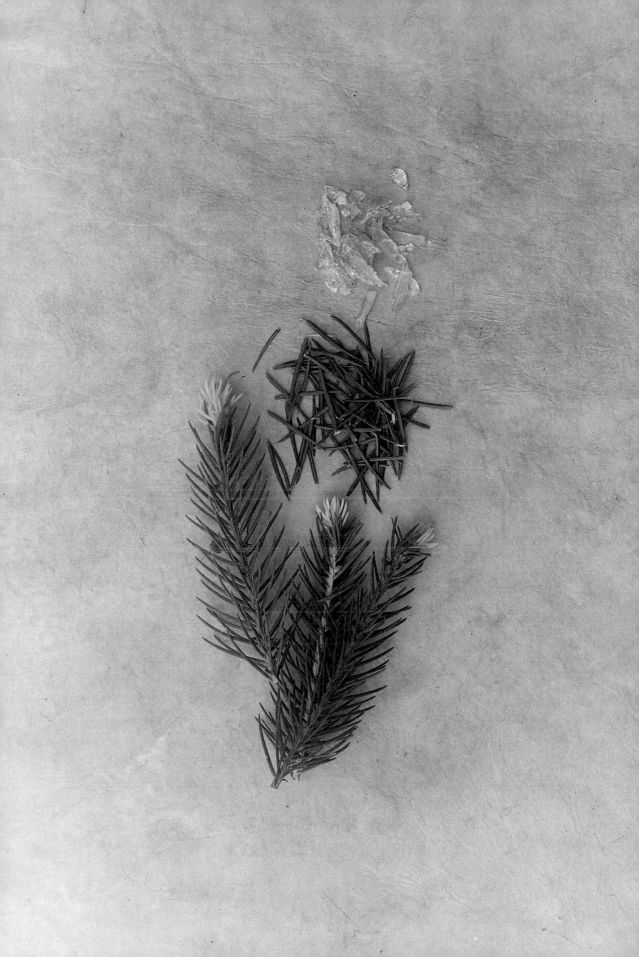

Stinging Nettle

Urtica dioica

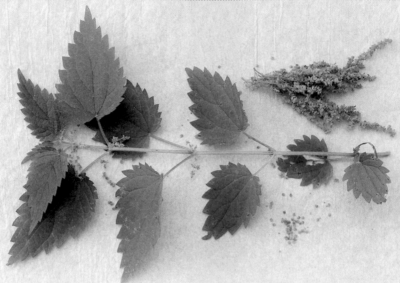

Where Does It Grow?

Virtually everywhere in the world.

What Does It Look Like?

A frost-hardy herbaceous perennial that grows up to 5 feet (1.5 m) tall, stinging nettle has heavily toothed leaves. Except for the young shoots, which appear from March to May, the entire plant is covered with tiny stinging hairs. The greenish-white flower clusters appear between May and July.

Which Parts Are Used?

The leaves and seeds.

What Does It Do?

The stinging nettle has a purifying and detoxifying effect. In addition, it contains anti-inflammatory and analgesic substances, which make it indispensable in the treatment of rheumatism and arthritis. It is also indicated for bladder and urinary tract problems, as well as prostate disorders.

How Can I Use It?

Spring Tea (page 95), Virility Tea (page 126), Hair Tonic (page 127) and Nettle Wine (page 128). To make nettle tea, which has the same effect as Nettle Wine without the alcohol, place 3 to 4 tsp (15 to 20 mL) fresh nettle leaves (or 1 tsp/5 mL dried) in a cup, pour a generous $\frac{3}{4}$ cup (200 mL) boiling water over top, then cover and let steep for 10 minutes.

What Do Scientists Think of It?

Numerous clinical studies with tens of thousands of participants have proven the efficacy of the stinging nettle plant. Studies of people with rheumatic diseases showed that more than half of them experienced less pain when using stinging nettle extract. Men with enlarged prostates who used stinging nettle extract reported that their need to urinate during the night was reduced by half; and that their urine flow increased and the amount of urine retained in the bladder decreased.

Sweet Violet

Viola odorata

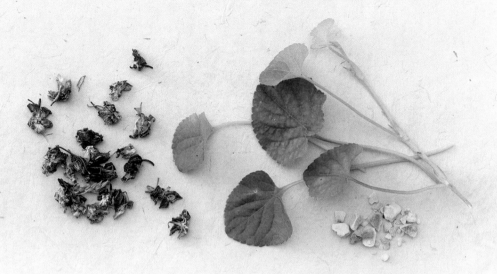

Where Does It Grow?
Europe and Asia.

What Does It Look Like?
Sweet violet is a small, usually perennial plant with a frost-hardy rootstock that spreads from year to year. The short-stemmed, dark green leaves are at times divided and toothed along the margins. Many violet-colored, pleasantly scented flowers appear from March to April.

Which Parts Are Used?
The flowering herb and the root.

What Does It Do?
In ancient times, sweet violets were used to treat headaches and poor vision. Today, the plant is often one of the ingredients in cough linctus (better known as cough syrup in North America) because it has an expectorant effect. Sweet violets are also highly esteemed for their blood-cleansing properties.

How Can I Use It?
Irritable Cough Tea (page 76).

What Do Scientists Think of It?
In 2009, scientists at the University of Bochum, Germany, were able to demonstrate (in test tube studies) that the scent of the sweet violet flower can inhibit the growth of prostate cancer cells. Further studies are needed to show whether this might be the starting point for developing a future therapy.

Caution
Do not confuse sweet violet with the violet root that is sold in pharmacies and organic stores as a natural teething aid for babies. Violet root bears no relation to the sweet violet; it is actually an iris rhizome.

Tea Tree

Melaleuca alternifolia

Where Does It Grow?
Australia.

What Does It Look Like?
The tea tree is an evergreen shrub or small tree that grows up to 23 to 33 feet (7 to 10 m) tall, with white bark. Young branches are wooly; older ones are hairless. The tiny yellow or cream-colored flowers appear in spring. The narrow, lance-shaped leaves contain numerous glands; these exude tea tree oil.

Which Parts Are Used?
The essential oil distilled from the leaves and young shoots.

What Does It Do?
People in Australia have used tea tree oil as a disinfectant for wounds since prehistoric times. Today, the oil is also used to treat acne, skin rashes, bad breath and athlete's foot.

How Can I Use It?
Gargling Solution (page 72) and Tea Tree Oil Mouthwash (page 145).

What Do Scientists Think of It?
In several studies, scientists have been able to confirm the bactericidal and fungicidal properties of tea tree oil.

Caution
There is no scientific evidence on the effects of tea tree oil use on pregnant or breastfeeding women; it is best to refrain from using it during those times. People who suffer from allergies should test the oil on a small area of skin to gauge their reaction before using tea tree oil. Never use tea tree oil internally, and always store it out of the reach of children.

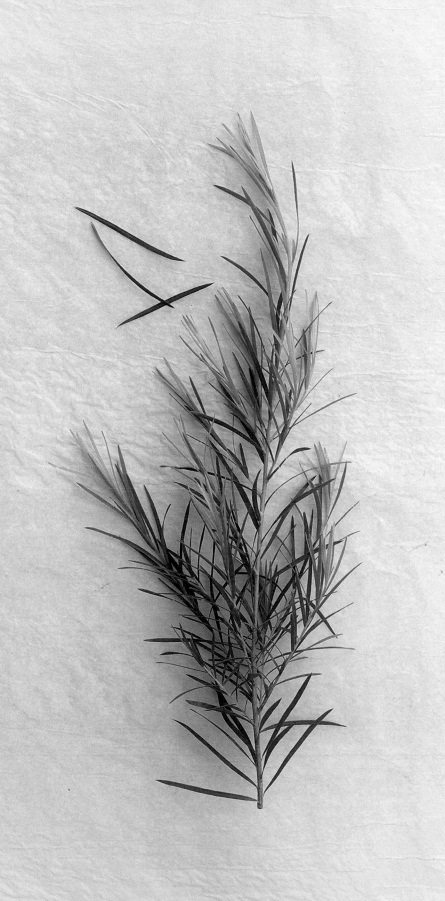

Thyme

Thymus vulgaris

Where Does It Grow?
Originally native to the Mediterranean region; today, cultivated widely all around the world.

What Does It Look Like?
A perennial, usually partly wooded, dwarf shrub, thyme grows up to 20 inches (50 cm) tall. Small, oval leaflets rise from the hairy stems, often curled downward. The leaflets are gray-green on top; lighter in color on the downy undersides. Blue-violet to light red flowers appear from April to September. The entire plant exudes an intense aroma.

Which Parts Are Used?
The leaves and flowers, fresh or dried.

What Does It Do?
Thyme essential oil (also called thymol) has expectorant and bactericidal properties, and promotes the evacuation of phlegm. This is why the plant is often used to treat bronchitis and whooping cough. Thyme also stimulates digestion and helps the body tolerate fatty foods.

How Can I Use It?
Irritable Cough Tea (page 76), Thyme Cream (page 80) and Love Liqueur (page 124). To make a simple thyme tea, place 1 tsp (5 mL) thyme leaves in a cup, pour a generous ¾ cup (200 mL) boiling water over top, then cover and let steep for 10 minutes.

What Do Scientists Think of It?
Thyme has been well researched, and its antibiotic, antiviral and fungicidal actions have been documented in multiple laboratory tests. Thus, the German Commission E and the European agency ESCOP (see page 155) recommend thyme for inflammations of the respiratory tract, bronchitis and whooping cough. In addition, ESCOP endorses thyme for the treatment of inflamed stomach linings and as a remedy against bad breath.

Caution
Consult your doctor or midwife before using thyme if you are pregnant or breastfeeding. The herb supposedly stimulates the contraction of the uterus, although this conclusion is controversial.

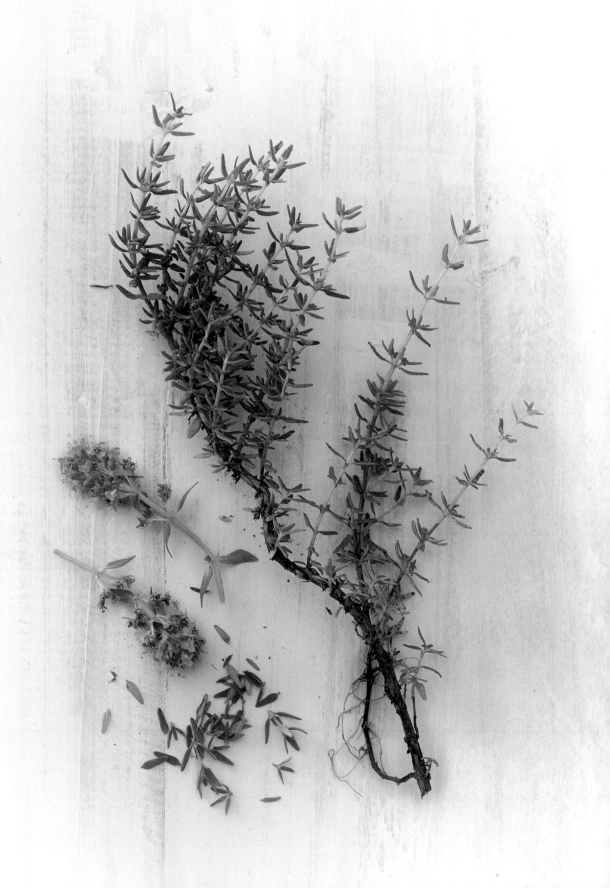

Tormentil (Bloodroot)

Potentilla erecta

Where Does It Grow?

Europe, North Africa, western Siberia and North America.

What Does It Look Like?

An herbaceous perennial that grows about 12 inches (30 cm) tall, tormentil has widely branched stalks and feathery leaves. The small, intensely yellow, four-petaled flowers appear from March to June. The rhizomes are harvested in the spring and the fall.

Which Parts Are Used?

The rhizome.

What Does It Do?

Tormentil is also known as bloodroot. The name was coined both because of the dark red sap that the root exudes when cut and because of its ability to stop hemorrhages. Tormentil is used externally on slow-healing wounds, frostbite, burns, and wounds and inflammations of the mucous membranes of the mouth and throat. It is also used to treat pressure points caused by dentures; in this case, rinse your mouth several times a day with tormentil tea.

Used internally, tormentil also has contracting and analgesic properties. It also has a constipating effect, which is helpful in the case of diarrhea.

How Can I Use It?

Tormentil Tea (page 42).

What Do Scientists Think of It?

The German Commission E (see page 155) endorses the administration of tormentil in cases of acute diarrhea and minor inflammations of the mouth and throat.

Caution

When tormentil is taken over a long period of time or in high doses, it may cause damage to the liver or kidneys. Pregnant and breastfeeding women should consult their physician or natural health practitioner before using tormentil, because there is not sufficient scientific evidence on its use during these times.

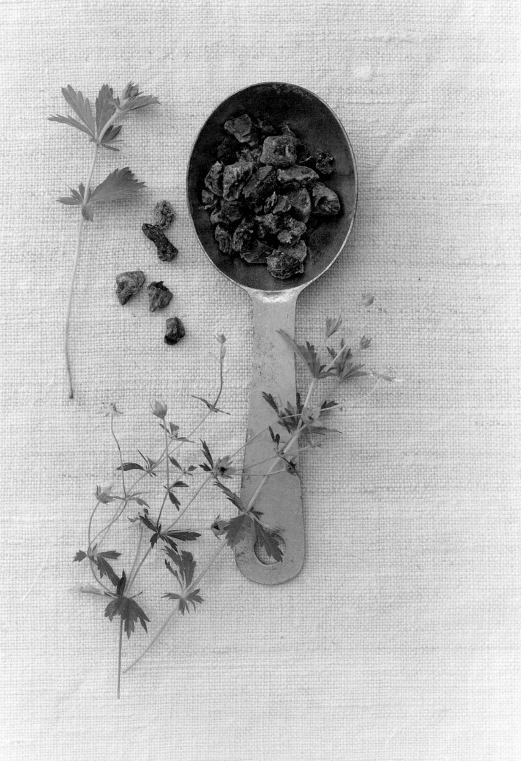

Valerian

Valeriana officinalis

Where Does It Grow?

Europe and Asia.

What Does It Look Like?

Valerian is a hardy perennial plant that grows up to 3 feet (1 m) tall, with leaves that get progressively smaller toward the top. White or pink umbels of flowers appear throughout the summer. The roots are harvested in the fall.

Which Parts Are Used?

The roots and the flowers.

What Does It Do?

The ideal plant remedy for anxiety, nervousness, irritability and insomnia, valerian makes it easier to fall asleep and improves the quality of sleep.

How Can I Use It?

Heart and Nerve Tonic (page 84). For anxiety, make a simple tea: place 1 tsp (5 mL) dried valerian root in a cup, pour a generous ¾ cup (200 mL) boiling water over top, then cover and let steep for 10 minutes.

What Do Scientists Think of It?

Numerous studies have been able to demonstrate scientifically that valerian improves quality of sleep, that users felt better rested after waking up and that their general well-being was improved. The German Commission E and the European agency ESCOP (see page 155) endorse the use of valerian for nervous sleep disorders and anxiety.

Caution

In order for valerian to achieve its full effect, you should use the preparation for a minimum of four weeks. But be cautious: one to two hours after taking the remedy, your ability to react may be diminished. You should not drive a car or operate heavy machinery if you have taken a valerian preparation. Because there is a lack of scientific evidence on the use of valerian during pregnancy, you should refrain from using it during that time.

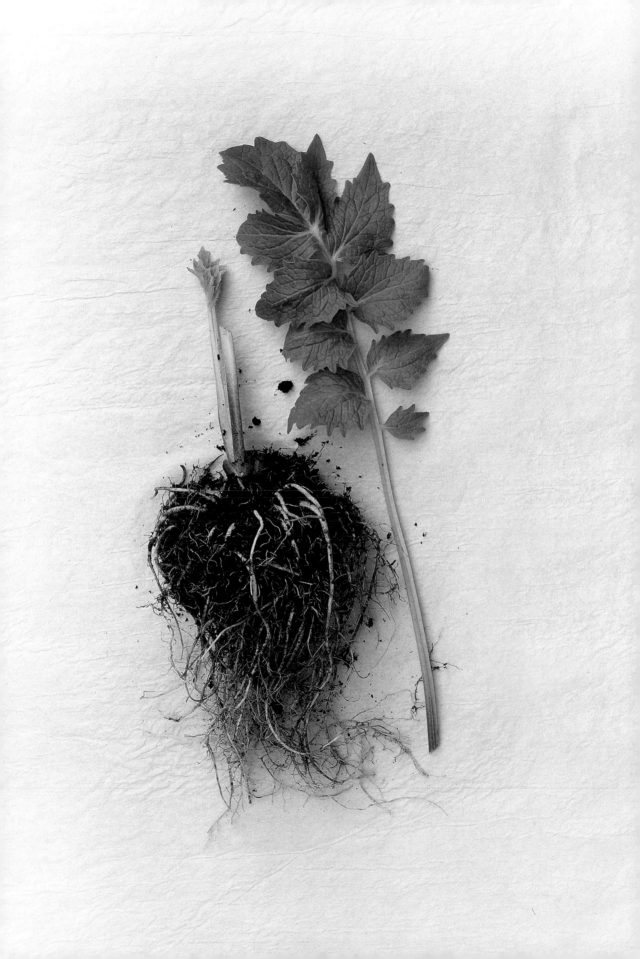

Yarrow

Achillea millefolium

Where Does It Grow?

Europe and temperate parts of Asia.

What Does It Look Like?

Yarrow is an herbaceous, perennial plant that grows up to 28 inches (70 cm) tall, with elongated, highly feathered leaves. Between May and October, small white or light pink flowers form in loose heads on top of the upright hairy stems.

Which Parts Are Used?

The whole plant, especially the flowers.

What Does It Do?

Yarrow was once also known as "stanchweed" because that's exactly what it does: it helps stop (stanch) bleeding. This property, combined with yarrow's anti-inflammatory substances, makes the herb unbeatable in the battle against hemorrhoids. In addition, the plant is antispasmodic, helps treat digestive disorders and is believed to alleviate menopausal complaints.

Yarrow can also be used to treat pimples. First, make a simple yarrow tea: place 1 tsp (5 mL) yarrow flowers in a cup, pour a generous ¾ cup (200 mL) boiling water over top, then cover and let steep for 10 minutes. Dip a cloth into the tea, gently squeeze the liquid out and place on top of the inflamed area.

How Can I Use It?

Chasteberry Healing Vinegar (page 106), Yarrow Balm (page 120) and Bitters (page 146).

What Do Scientists Think of It?

It has not yet been possible to scientifically verify the antispasmodic and anti-inflammatory qualities of yarrow, but the German Commission E (see page 155) recommends taking the herb internally for lack of appetite and applying it externally (such as in a sitz bath) for functional lower abdomen problems in women, such as irritable bowel syndrome.

Caution

If you are allergic to daisies or other similar flowers, test the yarrow preparation on a small area of skin before using or consuming it.

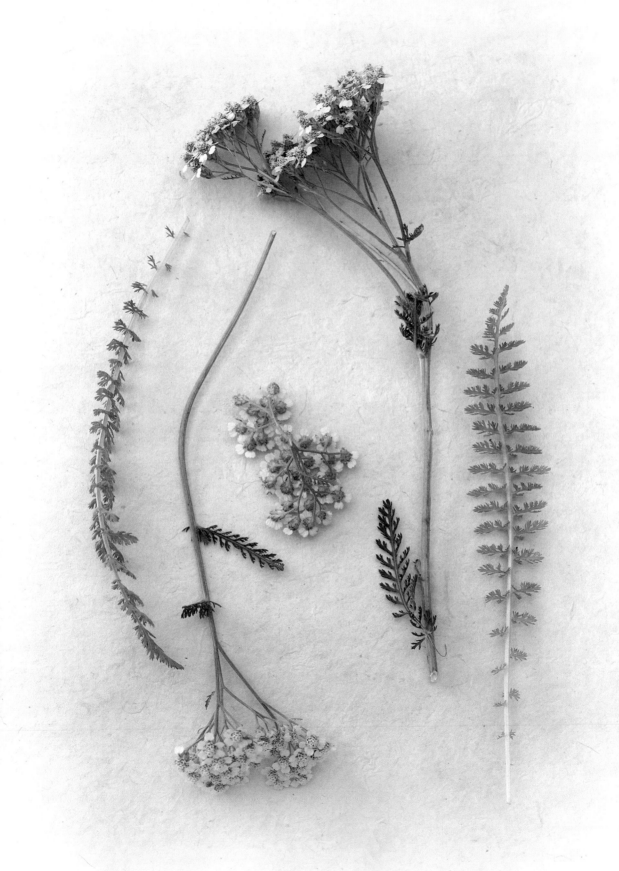

Yellow Gentian

Gentiana lutea

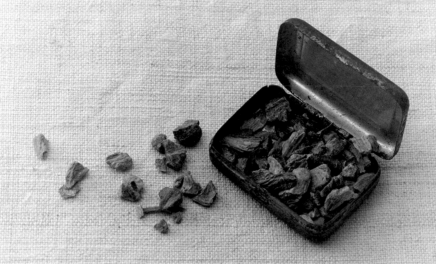

Where Does It Grow?

Originally a native of the mountainous regions of central and southern Europe; today, it is widely cultivated around the world.

What Does It Look Like?

Yellow gentian is a perennial herb, which grows up to 5 feet (1.5 m) tall and has a thick root that can grow to 3 feet (1 m) long. The large oval leaves form a ground-hugging rosette; they have several pronounced arched veins. The long-stemmed, bright yellow flowers, which have five sepals, appear from June to August.

Which Parts Are Used?

The root.

What Does It Do?

Yellow gentian contains many bitter substances that boost bowel and digestive system activity. It is therefore used to treat flatulence, stomach complaints and digestive disorders. In combination with cowslip flowers, sorrel, elder flowers and verbena (usually in the form of capsules or drops), it has proved successful in treating sinus inflammation. Because of its bitter taste, yellow gentian is always combined with other herbs.

How Can I Use It?

Healing Vinegar (page 85).

What Do Scientists Think of It?

Scientists have not yet studied the effects of yellow gentian.

Caution

Gentian should not be taken during pregnancy or while breastfeeding, because there is a lack of evidence on its use during these times.

Other Medicinal Herbs Used in the Recipes

Angelica (*Angelica* spp.)
- **Where It Grows:** Northern and eastern Europe, Siberia, Himalayas and North America.
- **What It Looks Like:** Deciduous plant, flowers only once, 3 to 10 feet (1 to 3 m) tall, with numerous flowers grouped into large umbels.
- **What It Does:** Boosts immunity, antiseptic, sedative, cleanses the blood, promotes blood flow, strengthens the heart, antispasmodic, tonifying.
- **Ingredient in:** Virility Tea (page 126).

Chamomile (*Matricaria chamomilla*)
- **Where It Grows:** Europe, North America and Australia.
- **What It Looks Like:** Strongly scented herb, 6 to 20 inches (15 to 50 cm) tall, with many white-yellow flower heads.
- **What It Does:** Analgesic, antispasmodic and antiseptic; soothes body, mind and spirit.
- **Ingredient in:** Bentonite Clay Face Mask (page 56).

Chasteberry (*Vitex agnus-castus*)
- **Where It Grows:** The entire Mediterranean region, temperate climatic zones of Asia.
- **What It Looks Like:** Shrub, up to 13 feet (4 m) tall, with hand-shaped, feathered leaves and white, pink or violet flower clusters.
- **What It Does:** Helps treat premenstrual syndrome (PMS), menstrual cycle disorders, inability to conceive, inflammations of the testicles or the prostate, and hyperexcitability.
- **Ingredient in:** Chasteberry Healing Vinegar (page 106).

Cinnamon (*Cinnamomum* spp.)
- **Where It Grows:** Southern Asia.
- **What It Looks Like:** Dried bark of the cinnamon tree; available as cinnamon sticks or ground cinnamon.
- **What It Does:** Antibacterial, antispasmodic, expectorant, analgesic, tonifying, warming; lowers blood sugar.
- **Ingredient in:** Love Liqueur (page 124).

Echinacea or Purple Coneflower (*Echinacea* spp.)
- **Where It Grows:** North America.
- **What It Looks Like:** An herbaceous flowering plant in the daisy family, with large orange to purple flower heads.
- **What It Does:** Supportive for respiratory and urinary infections; used externally for slow-healing wounds.
- **Ingredient in:** Sinus Tea (page 77).

Iceland Moss (*Cetraria islandica*)
- **Where It Grows:** Arctic regions, heathland, moors and coniferous forests.
- **What It Looks Like:** Lichen species, $1\frac{1}{2}$ to $4\frac{3}{4}$ inches (4 to 12 cm) tall, with leaf-like, curved or tube-like rolled-in shoots that are brownish-green on top and white-green underneath.
- **What It Does:** Strengthens mucous membranes; antibacterial, soothing, invigorating, tonifying.
- **Ingredient in:** Irritable Cough Tea (page 76).

Juniper Berries (*Juniperus communis*)
- **Where It Grows:** Europe, northern Asia and North America.
- **What It Looks Like:** Pillar-shaped shrub that yields medicinal berries.

- **What It Does:** Antibacterial and analgesic; hematopoietic (blood forming) and blood cleansing; acts as a diuretic, expectorant and diaphoretic (induces perspiration); tonifying.
- **Ingredient in:** Bitters (page 146).

Lady's Mantle (*Alchemilla* spp.)
- **Where It Grows:** Europe, Asia and Africa.
- **What It Looks Like:** Tender plant with cup-shaped, lobed leaves and pale yellow flower panicles.
- **What It Does:** Astringent, styptic, blood cleansing, antispasmodic, tonifying, diuretic.
- **Ingredient in:** Chasteberry Healing Vinegar (page 106).

Licorice (*Glycyrrhiza* spp.)
- **Where It Grows:** Subtropical regions of Europe and Asia.
- **What It Looks Like:** Perennial plant that grows up to $6\frac{1}{2}$ feet (2 m) tall; the root is used medicinally.
- **What It Does:** Fights coughs, stomach ulcers, headaches and low blood pressure; cleanses the blood.
- **Ingredient in:** Irritable Cough Tea (page 76).

Lovage (*Levisticum officinale*)
- **Where It Grows:** The entire Mediterranean region.
- **What It Looks Like:** Member of the carrot family, up to $6\frac{1}{2}$ feet (2 m) tall.

- **What It Does:** Stimulating, diaphoretic, antispasmodic, styptic, diuretic, boosts metabolism, anti-inflammatory.
- **Ingredient in:** Virility Tea (page 126).

Mace (*Myristica* spp.)
- **Where It Grows:** Europe and large parts of Asia.
- **What It Looks Like:** Large tree that produces a seed we call nutmeg; mace is the red, net-like covering of the nutmeg kernel.
- **What It Does:** Stimulating, astringent, calming, antispasmodic.
- **Ingredient in:** Love Liqueur (page 124).

Marshmallow (*Althaea officinalis*)
- **Where It Grows:** Southeastern Europe and western Asia.
- **What It Looks Like:** Member of the mallow family, up to 5 feet (1.5 m) tall, with light pink flowers.
- **What It Does:** Calms irritated mucous membranes in the throat during colds, dry coughs and hoarseness.
- **Ingredient in:** Irritable Cough Tea (page 76).

Mullein (*Verbascum* spp.)
- **Where It Grows:** Europe and northern Asia.
- **What It Looks Like:** Plant that grows up to $6\frac{1}{2}$ feet (2 m) tall, with a bolt-upright stem; ground-hugging leaf rosette, bright yellow flowers.

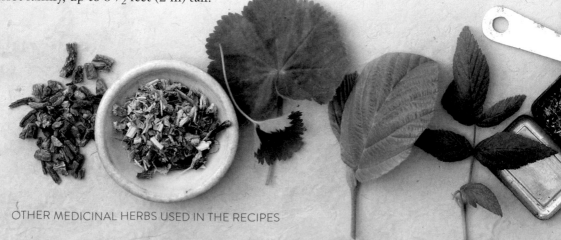

- **What It Does:** Curative for bronchitis and coughs, asthma and infections of the gastrointestinal tract.
- **Ingredient in:** Expectorant Tea (page 75).

Myrtle *(Myrtus communis)*
- **Where It Grows:** The entire Mediterranean region, and the Canary Islands.
- **What It Looks Like:** Strongly branched evergreen shrub, up to 16 feet (5 m) tall, with numerous white flowers.
- **What It Does:** Promotes secretion; enhances appetite.
- **Ingredient in:** Sinus Tea (page 77).

Peppermint *(Mentha x piperita)*
- **Where It Grows:** Throughout the world, in all temperate zones.
- **What It Looks Like:** Frost-hardy plant with oval, serrated leaves and violet inflorescences; the entire plant exudes an intense aroma.
- **What It Does:** Antimicrobial, antispasmodic and antiviral; acts as an expectorant, stimulates digestion and purges bile; sedative.
- **Ingredient in:** Sinus Tea (page 77).

Red Raspberry Leaf *(Rubus idaeus)*
- **Where It Grows:** Europe and the temperate climate zone of Asia.

- **What It Looks Like:** Deciduous shrub, up to 6 1/2 feet (2 m) tall, flowers from May to June.
- **What It Does:** Relaxes the muscles of the uterus and the digestive tract.
- **Ingredient in:** Yarrow Balm (page 120).

Rhubarb Root *(Rhei radix)*
- **Where It Grows:** Tibet and China.
- **What It Looks Like:** Root of a perennial plant, *Rheum rhabarbarum,* with up to 5-foot (1.5 m) tall stems and large, round to heart-shaped leaves.
- **What It Does:** Stimulates elimination, promotes colonic motility.
- **Ingredient in:** Bitters (page 146).

Ribwort Plantain *(Plantago lanceolata)*
- **Where It Grows:** Europe and parts of Asia.
- **What It Looks Like:** A perennial plant with ground-hugging rosettes of leaves; an inconspicuous flower spike rises from the long stem.
- **What It Does:** Antibacterial and anti-inflammatory; cleanses the blood and stanches bleeding; acts as a diuretic and expectorant; astringent.
- **Ingredient in:** Irritable Cough Tea (page 76).

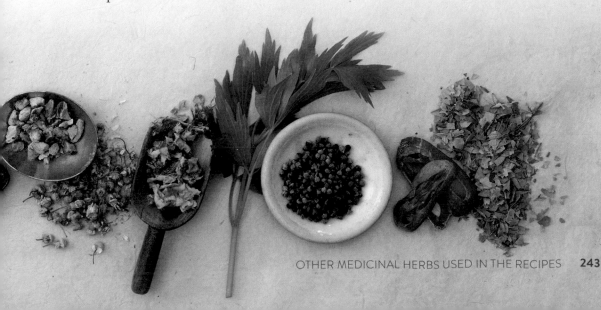

Senna (*Senna alexandrina*)
- **Where It Grows:** Africa and the Middle East.
- **What It Looks Like:** A shrub, 20 inches to 5 feet (50 cm to 1.5 m) tall, with feathered foliage and bright yellow flower racemes.
- **What It Does:** Proven treatment for constipation and hemorrhoids; soothes after rectal surgery; cleanses and evacuates the intestines.
- **Ingredient in:** Fig Syrup (page 142).

Sweet Flag or Calamus Root (*Acorus calamus*)
- **Where It Grows:** Originally Eastern Asia; today, grown in Asia, North America, and central and eastern Europe.
- **What It Looks Like:** Reed, up to 5 feet (1.5 m) tall, with brownish-yellow spikes.
- **What It Does:** Antispasmodic in the gastrointestinal tract; helps fight flatulence and constipation; helps treat bronchitis, toothache, insomnia and depression.
- **Ingredient in:** Bitters (page 146).

Vanilla (*Vanilla planifolia*)
- **Where It Grows:** Native of Mexico; today, found in zones all around the equator.
- **What It Looks Like:** Edible flower of a climbing orchid, up to 33 feet (10 m) tall.
- **What It Does:** Boosts physical and mental performance; improves mood; alleviates anxiety, fatigue and depressive moods; aphrodisiac.
- **Ingredient in:** Love Liqueur (page 124).

Walnut (*Juglans regia*)
- **Where It Grows:** Both temperate and subtropical climatic zones of the northern hemisphere.
- **What It Looks Like:** Fruit of the walnut tree; a tasty kernel is hidden by a hard, light brown shell, which itself sits inside a green husk.
- **What It Does:** Improves liver and heart function, blood vessels, skin problems and hair; is said to inhibit prostate cancer.
- **Ingredient in:** Hair Tonic (page 127).

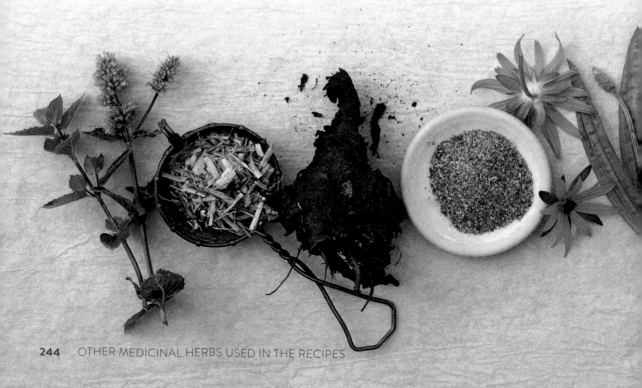

Wild Thyme (*Thymus* spp.)

- **Where It Grows:** Mediterranean region.
- **What It Looks Like:** Shrub, up to 12 inches (30 cm) tall, with numerous small oval leaves and violet flowers; also known as creeping thyme.
- **What It Does:** Fights respiratory diseases, digestive disorders, liver complaints, gallbladder diseases and colicky abdominal pains.
- **Ingredient in:** Expectorant Tea (page 75).

Witch Hazel (*Hamamelis* spp.)

- **Where It Grows:** All temperate areas of the northern hemisphere.
- **What It Looks Like:** Shrubs and small trees with gray-brown bark, with leathery leaves that are toothed along the margins; the flower buds appear on bare branches.
- **What It Does:** Styptic, anti-inflammatory; reduces itching.
- **Ingredient in:** Hair Tonic (page 127).

Wormwood (*Artemisia absinthium*)

- **Where It Grows:** Temperate parts of Eurasia, and North Africa.
- **What It Looks Like:** Perennial herbaceous plant, up to 24 inches (60 cm) tall, with feathered, gray-green leaves, densely covered in downy hairs on top, with aromatic small yellow flower heads.
- **What It Does:** Hematopoietic (fosters blood cell formation) and cleanses the blood; helps fight indigestion and flatulence.
- **Ingredient in:** Bitters (page 146).

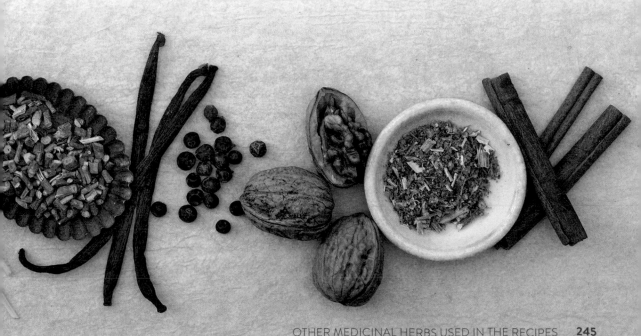

Resources

Organizations and Information

American Herbal Products Association
8630 Fenton St., Suite 918
Silver Spring, MD 20910, U.S.A.
www.ahpa.org
*A national trade association focused on herbs,
botanicals and herbal products.*

American Herbalists Guild
125 South Lexington Ave., Suite 101
Asheville, NC 28801, U.S.A.
www.americanherbalistsguild.com
*A nonprofit, educational organization that
represents herbalists specializing in the medicinal
use of plants.*

Canadian Council of Herbalist Associations
362 Rue Sainte-Catherine
Longueuil, QC J4H 2C1, Canada
http://herbalccha.org
*A nonprofit organization representing
associations of herbal practitioners through
communication with government, with the
public, and between all herbalist associations
in Canada.*

Canadian Organic Growers
National Office
1145 Carling Ave., Suite 7519
Ottawa, ON K1Z 7K4, Canada
www.cog.ca
*Canada's national information network for
organic farmers, gardeners and consumers.*

European Scientific Cooperative on
Phytotherapy (ESCOP)
Notaries House
Chapel Street
Exeter, Devon EX1 1EZ, U.K.
www.escop.com
*An umbrella organization representing
national phytotherapy associations across Europe.*

Herb Society of America
9019 Kirtland Chardon Rd.
Kirtland, OH 44094, U.S.A.
www.herbsociety.org
*A national organization that educates
its members and the public on the cultivation
of herbs, and their history and uses, both past
and present.*

International Herb Association
P.O. Box 5667
Jacksonville, FL 32247-5667, U.S.A.
www.iherb.org
*A trade association that specializes in
educational, service and development opportunities
for herbal professionals who are growing,
marketing and using herbs.*

National Herbalists Association of Australia
4 Cavendish St.
Concord West, NSW 2138, Australia
www.nhaa.org.au
*A national professional association of western
herbalists and naturopaths.*

National Institute of Medical Herbalists
Clover House
James Court
South Street
Exeter, Devon EX1 1EE, U.K.
www.nimh.org.uk
*The United Kingdom's leading professional body
representing herbal practitioners.*

Saskatchewan Herb and Spice Association
P.O. Box 7568, Station Main
Saskatoon, SK S7K 4L4, Canada
www.saskherbspice.org
*The secretariat for the Canadian Herb, Spice
and Natural Health Product Coalition, a
national coalition working to create a profitable,
sustainable Canadian herb, spice and natural
health product industry.*

Products

Abundant Health
222 W. 3560 N.
Spanish Fork, UT 84660, U.S.A.
www.abundanthealth4u.com
Glass and plastic bottles, specialty containers, funnels and jars.

Bottles.com
1521 Cades Bay
Jupiter, FL 33458, U.S.A.
www.ebottles.com
Glass and plastic bottles, canning and cosmetic jars, spray and roll-on bottles.

Bulk Herb Store
26 West 6th Ave.
Lobelville, TN 37097, U.S.A.
www.bulkherbstore.com
Bulk herbs, herbal mixes and tinctures.

Elk Mountain Herbs
214 Ord St.
Laramie, WY 82070, U.S.A.
www.elkmountainherbs.com
Tinctures, bulk herbs, teas and ceremonial herbs.

1st Chinese Herbs
5018 Viewridge Dr.
Olympia, WA 98501, U.S.A.
www.1stchineseherbs.com
Bulk herbs for traditional Chinese medicine, extracts, and ready-made creams and ointments.

Gaia Herbs
101 Gaia Herbs Dr.
Brevard, NC 28712, U.S.A.
www.gaiaherbs.com
Herbal extracts, teas and supplements.

Healing Spirits Herb Farm
61247 Route 415
Avoca, NY 14809, U.S.A.
www.healingspiritsherbfarm.com
Bulk herbs, tinctures, extracts, oils, teas and ready-made herbal cosmetics.

The Herbalist
2106 NE 65th St.
Seattle, WA 98115, U.S.A.
http://store.theherbalist.com
Bulk herbs, essential oils, herb extracts and ready-made remedies.

Herb Pharm
P.O. Box 116
Williams, OR 97544, U.S.A.
www.herb-pharm.com
Herb oils and liquid extracts, capsules and powders.

Hollow Reed Holistic
3-875 Corydon Ave.
Winnipeg, MB R3M 0W7, Canada
www.hollowreedholistic.ca
Bulk herbs, essential oils, homeopathic remedies and tinctures.

Horizon Herbs
P.O. Box 69
Williams, OR 97544, U.S.A.
www.horizonherbs.com
Bulk herbs, extracts, seeds and plants.

Judy's Organic Herbs
P.O. Box 258
Woodlawn, ON K0A 3M0, Canada
www.earthmedicine.ca
Bulk and Ayurvedic herbs, tinctures, teas and ready-made remedies.

Mountain Rose Herbs
P.O. Box 50220
Eugene, OR 97405, U.S.A.
www.mountainroseherbs.com
Bulk herbs, teas, essential and other oils, containers and ready-made remedies.

Pacific Botanicals
4840 Fish Hatchery Rd.
Grants Pass, OR 97527, U.S.A.
www.pacificbotanicals.com
Bulk and Ayurvedic herbs, containers, herb seeds and seaweeds.

Richters
357 Hwy 47
Goodwood, ON L0C 1A0, Canada
www.richters.com
Bulk herbs, essential oils, seeds and plants.

Saffire Blue
1444 Bell Mill Rd.
Tillsonburg, ON N4G 4G9, Canada
www.saffireblue.ca
Glass and plastic bottles, jars, vegetable oils and essential oils.

Sage Woman Herbs
108 E. Cheyenne Rd.
Colorado Springs, CO 80906, U.S.A.
www.sagewomanherbs.com
Bulk herbs, capsules, essential oils, tinctures, supplements and teas.

Salt Spring Seeds
Box 444, Ganges P.O.
Salt Spring Island, BC V8K 2W1, Canada
www.saltspringseeds.com
Organic heirloom medicinal herb seeds.

Specialty Bottle
3434 4th Ave. S.
Seattle, WA 98134, U.S.A.
www.specialtybottle.com
Glass bottles and jars, plastic bottles and jars, and tins.

SKS Bottle & Packaging, Inc.
2600 7th Ave.
Building 60 West
Watervliet, NY 12189, U.S.A.
www.sks-bottle.com
Glass, plastic and specialty bottles; jars; labels; and tins.

Woodland Essence
392 Teacup St.
Cold Brook, NY 13324, U.S.A.
www.woodlandessence.com
Flower essences, massage oils, creams and extracts.

Zack Woods Herb Farm
278 Mead Rd.
Hyde Park, VT 05655, U.S.A.
www.zackwoodsherbs.com
Bulk herbs, teas and plants.

Library and Archives Canada Cataloguing in Publication

Wenzel, Melanie
[Meine besten heilpflanzenrezepte. English]
        The essential guide to home herbal remedies : easy
recipes using medicinal herbs to treat more than 125 conditions
from sunburns to sore throats / Melanie Wenzel.

Includes index.
Translation of: Meine besten Heilpflanzenrezepte.
ISBN 978-0-7788-0489-5 (pbk.)

        1. Herbs--Therapeutic use--Popular works. I. Title.
III. Title: Meine besten heilpflanzenrezepte. English

RM666.H33W4513 2014   615.3'21   C2014-903340-0

Index